Praise for *The Final Journey*

"Sangita's book is compassionate, practical, and wise—Krishna conscious."

—Giriraj Swami

"'If someone is physically, emotionally, and mentally pain free, has other symptoms well managed, and is rightly situated spiritually, he will experience an auspicious, most glorious passing away.' So affirms Susan Pattinson, RN (Sangita Devi Dasi) in *The Final Journey—Complete Hospice Care for Departing Vaishnavas*, where she gives relevant information for the care of the dying gained from years of practice as a hospice nurse and practice of *sadhana bhakti* under Srila Prabhupada, her spiritual master. Indeed, the book is a veritable 'gold mine' of valuable information. Her presentation, showing how the aforesaid can be realized, is exhaustive and profoundly sensitive. Painstakingly she indicates how hospice care for certain terminally ill can facilitate that glorious death for which all Vaishnavas aspire."

—The late Sarah Caner Schofield, Ph.D. (Saranagati Devi Dasi), Former Director of Volunteers, Albert Einstein Medical Center Hospice

"Death is a prominent subject matter in Krishna conscious philosophy, since it is our chance to go back to Godhead. Yet, the actual process of dying is an uncomfortable topic that we tend to keep at a respectful distance. *The Final Journey—Complete Hospice Care for Departing Vaishnavas* is the first of its kind in ISKCON. It is a much-needed, simple, and practical guide to care of the terminally ill from a Vaishnava perspective. Drawing on the author's extensive experience as a hospice registered nurse, the book provides a wealth of detailed information. The author's area of expertise is allopathic pain management for the terminally ill, and she argues convincingly that a drug's long-term effect on a dying body is moot, while greater comfort increases the ability to hear and chant. Alternatives are provided as well. This book takes the reader step-by-step through the entire process, and there is no doubt that it is an invaluable resource for everyone."

—Dharini Dasi, M.A. Applied Sociology, Attorney at Law

"I had the distinct pleasure of reading *The Final Journey—Complete Hospice Care for Departing Vaishnavas*. I found it very simple, informative, and appropriate for both devotees and non-devotees alike. As a Hospice Physician and Medical Director, I strongly recommend this book to families of terminally ill patients as well as to hospice professionals."

—Dr. Thiruvalam P. Indira, M.D.

"During his final days in Vrindavan in 1977, Srila Prabhupada told his disciples, 'Don't think this won't happen to you.' In light of this instruction, I highly recommend this book as a most important contribution to our society."

—Srutakirti Das, Srila Prabhupada's personal servant, 1972-75

"*The Final Journey—Complete Hospice Care for Departing Vaishnavas* provides the reader with extensive, palliative guidelines for the delivery of care to devotees in the last stages of life. This book is a textbook template for caring for the dying. Using comfortable vocabulary and real examples from her own life, the author provides us with a sense of confidence to take on this most glorious service—attending to Vaishnavas during the most important phase of their lives. As a nurse, I found this manual can serve as a resource for any person, regardless of skill set. As a devotee, I see that this can cross denominations and be applied to any soul preparing to leave his body."

—Brian O'Dea, RN, BSN

"It was a delight to read *The Final Journey—Complete Hospice Care for Departing Vaishnavas* by Susan Pattinson, RN (Sangita Devi Dasi) for three reasons. First, her obvious professional knowledge and experience in hospice care make this book a serious presentation on the subject. Thus it will serve as a practical tool for all concerned, as well as a reminder of how sensitive and qualified one should be for this service. Then, departing spiritualists can derive great benefit from modern medicine as it is applied to hospice care. As a spiritualist herself, the author also gives us inspiring and useful insights on the importance of a good death. She goes deep into subjects like compassion toward spiritual pain, respect for one's spiritual desires and convictions, importance of prayers and holy association, and relevant scriptural quotes. Finally, this book offers great hope to the aging Vaishnavas and will inspire members of our society to cooperate for this noble service of caring for others."

—Gopaswami Das (M.D., Qualified in Hospice Care)

"I'd like to commend you for publishing the excellent book '*The Final Journey*.' I've found it compassionate, thorough, professional, articulate, and obviously of great importance for Krishna conscious devotees. It's a great contribution, and you've done a great service by publishing it."

—Jayadvaita Swami

Sangita devi dasi delivers three intertwined books for the price of one. First, The Final Journey carefully depicts the natural dying process Second, Complete Hospice Care offers step-by-step – and eminently practical – guidance for terminal care. Third, the Departing Vaishnava addresses the spiritual and ritual needs of Chaitanya Vaishnavas, but – intriguingly – there is much here worth study by those of other faiths.. The Final Journey comes highly recommended to anyone who crosses paths with death.

—Robert Charles Powell, MD, PhD
Editorial Committee Member, Journal of Pastoral Care & Counseling
Past Member, COMISS Commission on Accreditation of Pastoral Services

The Final Journey

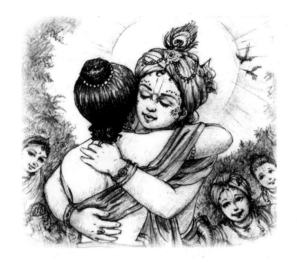

Complete Hospice Care for Departing Vaishnavas

Susan Pattinson, RN, CHPN
(Sangita Devi Dasi)

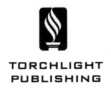

TORCHLIGHT PUBLISHING

Text copyright © 2002, 2011 (revised edition) by Susan Pattinson
Cover and internal illustrations copyright © 2011 by Deena Bandhu Das

All rights reserved. No part of this book may be reproduced, stored in a retrieval system, or transmitted in any form, by any means, including mechanical, electronic, photocopying, recording, or otherwise, without prior written consent of the publisher.

First Printing 2002
Second Printing 2011 Revised Edition

Cover and interior design by Manideep
Cover Illustration of Gopa Kumar and Krishna by Deena Bandhu Das
Printed in India
Published simultaneously in the United States and Canada by
Torchlight Publishing, Inc.

Library of Congress Cataloging-in-Publication Data

Pattinson, Susan, 1955-
 The final journey : complete hospice care for the departing Vaishnava / Susan Pattinson. -- 2nd rev. ed.
   p. ; cm.
 Includes bibliographical references.
 ISBN 978-0-9817273-9-4
 I. Title.
 [DNLM: 1. Hospice Care. 2. Hinduism. 3. Palliative Care. 4. Religion and Medicine. WB 310]

  362.17'560882945--dc23
                2011035093

Attention Colleges, Universities, Corporations, Associations, and Professional Organizations: The Final Journey is available at special discounts for bulk purchases for fund-raising or educational use. Special books, booklets, or excerpts can be created to suit your specific needs.

For more information, contact the Publisher:

Torchlight Publishing, Inc.
PO Box 52
Badger, CA 93603
Email: Torchlight@spiralcomm.net
Web: www.Torchlight.com

ACKNOWLEDGMENTS

I wish to express my sincere thanks to the following people who assisted with this book by providing their knowledge and spiritual insight: Padma Nabh Goswami, Indradyumna Swami, Bhakti Caru Swami, Deena Bandhu Das, Jananivas Das, and Kusha Devi Dasi.

Thank you to Jusaniya Devi Dasi for her tireless guidance, to Lalita-sakhi Devi Dasi for her expertise in editing this second edition of *The Final Journey*, and to Savitri Dasi for her exceptional proofreading, research, computer skills, and friendship.

My gratitude goes to His Holiness Giriraj Swami for his continuing support of this book and its goals. I also thank him for inspiring other Vaishnavas to participate in end-of-life care for those with terminal illnesses within this Krishna consciousness movement.

Many thanks to Advaita Candra Das (Alister Taylor), to whom I am deeply indebted for his continued encouragement and for being my publisher and mentor.

Our deep gratitude goes to Deena Bandhu Das for his inspirational drawing on the front cover and throughout the book.

Finally, my heartfelt appreciation goes to my husband Vamanadev Das, and our daughter Rajani, for their patience and support during the writing of this book.

Contents

Introduction..xv
What is Hospice?..1
   A History of the Hospice Movement 1
   Hospice and Palliative Care 2
   Experiencing a Terminal Illness 4
   Making the Decision 6
   Spiritual Care in Hospice 8
   The Dying Devotee's Bill of Rights 9
Practical Matters...11
   Who will Care for the Vaishnava? 11
   Where will the Vaishnava be Cared for? 14
   Should we Travel to the Holy Dhama? 18
   Choosing a Hospice in the West 19
   Living Wills 25
   A Living Will 26
   Medical Power of Attorney 28
What is Holistic Care?...39
   What is Spiritual Pain? 40
   How can the Caregiver Help? 41
   Communicating with One Who is Dying 45
Terminal Illnesses...51
   Acquired Immune Deficiency Syndrome (AIDS) 51
   Alzheimer's Disease 54
   Amyotrophic Lateral Sclerosis 55
   Cancer 56
   Cerebrovascular Disease (CVA) 58
   Chronic Obstructive Pulmonary Disease 59
   Congestive Heart Failure 59
   Diabetes Mellitus 60
   Hepatitis 61
   Multiple Sclerosis 65
   Parkinson's Disease 65

The Grief Process 67
    Denial 69
    Anger 71
    Bargaining 72
    Depression 73
    Acceptance 73
    When Young Children are Involved 74
    The Role of the Caregiver 77

Pain Management and the Use of Allopathic Medicine 78
    Pain Assessment 79
    A Word about Choices 81
    Three Major Analgesic Groups—Non-Opioid, Opioid,
    and Co-analgesics 81
    Dispelling the Myths 87
    Instant / Immediate Release Morphine 88
    Extended-Release Morphine Sulfate 89
    Dilaudid 91
    A Word about Using Demerol in Hospice Care 92
    Non-morphine Opioid 93
    Co-analgesics 94
    Commonly Used Co-analgesics and their Use in Hospice Care 95
    The World Health Organization Three Step Analgesic Ladder
    for Pain Control 98

Symptom Management 108
    Anorexia 108
    Anxiety 115
    Bleeding 118
    Constipation 122
    Diarrhea 125
    Dyspnea 127
    Edema 129
    Fever 132
    Nausea and Vomiting 136
    Dehydration versus Intravenous Fluid 139
    Physiology of the Terminally Ill Patient 140
    Benefits of Dehydration 140
    Difficulties Caused by Dehydration 141

Benefits of Intravenous Fluid 142
Detrimental Effects of Intravenous Fluid 143
PERSONAL CARE.. 145
Giving a Bed Bath 145
Washing your Patient's Hair 147
Changing a Bottom Sheet on an Occupied Bed 148
Using a Draw Sheet 148
Preventing Decubitus Ulcers (Pressure Sores) 149
What can be Done to Avoid Pressure Sores? 151
COMPLEMENTARY THERAPIES FOR COMFORT CARE........................ 154
Relaxation Techniques 154
Guided Imagery 155
Music Therapy 159
Aromatherapy 161
Some Suggested Essential Oils 164
Herbal Therapy 167
Cutaneous Stimulation/ Application of Heat and/ or Cold for
Pain Management 172
Therapeutic Massage for the Terminally Ill Patient 174
Basic Techniques 176
Srila Prabhupada's Remedies 178
Common Cold 178
Chest Cold and Congestion 179
Constipation 179
Diarrhea 179
Headache 179
Sore Muscles 179
Sore Throat 179
Stomach Ache Caused by Indigestion 180
Swollen Glands 180
Toothache 180
CARE OF THE CAREGIVER...181
Avoiding Caregiver Burnout 185
SIGNS AND SYMPTOMS OF APPROACHING DEATH......................... 187
Further Signs of Approaching Death 188
Decreased Eating and Drinking 190
Incontinence 191

    Vital Signs and Skin Color begin to Change 191
    Change in Breathing Pattern 192
    A Few Days to Hours before Death 193
    Assisting your Patient with Closure 195
    How do you Know when Death has Occurred? 200
POST-MORTEM CARE, CREMATION CEREMONY,
AND MEMORIAL SERVICE... 201
    Post-Mortem Care of the Vaishnava 201
    Cremation Ceremony in the West 202
    Memorial Service for the Vaishnava 203
    Remembering the Vaishnava 204
GRIEVING, HEALING, AND REJOICING FOR THE VAISHNAVA............... 206
    Understanding the Grief Reaction 208
    A Word about Excessive Grief 209
    A Word about Insufficient Grief 210
    The Tasks of the Bereaved and how We can Help.......................... 210
    Rejoicing for the Departed Vaishnava.. 213
    Additional Quotations from Srila Prabhupada 214
    Concluding Words 218
    PROCEDURE FOR PLACING ASHES IN THE YAMUNA RIVER................ 219
    PROCEDURE FOR PLACING ASHES IN THE GANGES RIVER................ 225
    PROCEDURE FOR SRADDHA CEREMONY.. 230

GLOSSARY... 234

BIBLIOGRAPHY... 248

INTRODUCTION

With the inevitable aging of the disciples of Srila Prabhupada, the Founder-*acarya* of the International Society for Krishna Consciousness (ISKCON) and later, his grand-disciples, the Bhaktivedanta Hospice was inaugurated in Vrindavan, India in 2010. For qualified Vaishnava doctors and nurses to care for devotees of Lord Krishna in the holy *dhama* is a most wonderful tribute to His Divine Grace. Serving those who are preparing for death encompasses all of the knowledge Srila Prabhupada gave us. Realistically, however, not everyone will be able to relocate to Vrindavan when diagnosed with a terminal illness. This does not mean that his or her passing away cannot be auspicious as well.

In the *Bhagavad-gita As It Is* (6.11-12), Srila Prabhupada writes:

'Sacred place' refers to places of pilgrimage. In India the *yogis*, transcendentalists, or the devotees, all leave home and reside in sacred places such as Prayaga, Mathura, Vrindavan, Hrsikesa, and Hardwar, and in solitude, practice yoga where the sacred rivers like the Yamuna and the Ganges flow. But, often this is not possible, especially for Westerners.... Therefore, in the *Brhan-Naradiya Purana* it is said that in *Kali-yuga* when people in general are short-lived, slow in spiritual realization, and always disturbed by various anxieties, the best means of spiritual realization is chanting the holy name of the Lord.

We can learn from this purport about the potency of chanting the Hare Krishna *maha-mantra* (*Hare Krishna Hare Krishna Krishna Krishna Hare Hare/Hare Rama Hare Rama Rama Rama Hare Hare*). When devotees face a terminal illness and are unable to travel to the holy *dhama*, chanting and hearing this transcendental sound vibration will transform any environment into a holy place. This was the gift given to us by Lord Chaitanya Mahaprabhu, the incarnation of Lord Krishna who appeared in India over 500 years ago to teach the method of achieving God-consciousness in this present age.—

To further establish this point, Srila Prabhupada writes in the *Bhagavad-gita* (8.15):

> The special qualification of the pure devotee is that he is always thinking of Krishna without considering the time or place. There should be no impediments. He should be able to carry out his service anywhere and at any time. Some say that the devotee should remain in holy places like Vrindavan or some holy town where the Lord lived, but a pure devotee can live anywhere and create the atmosphere of Vrindavan by his devotional service. It was Sri Advaita who told Lord Chaitanya, "Wherever You are, O Lord—there is Vrindavan."

Certainly I emphasize this point not to minimize the spiritual benefit of leaving one's body in the holy *dhama*. After all, Srila Prabhupada himself exemplified this importance when he traveled to Vrindavan to spend his final days. I simply wish to encourage those who are unable to do so and who now face the most significant challenge of their lives.

For those in need of this guide, it should be noted that it is not meant to replace a physician's advice or the care of a qualified hospice nurse. In the West, most hospices will send experienced nurses to the home for visits. If trained properly, they should be nonjudgmental and accepting of our spiritual beliefs. They should be able to work around our dietary needs as well as cooperate, if not appreciate, the importance of the patient wearing *tilak* (sacred clay markings), *tulasi* neckbeads, and having devotees present to chant and read scripture to the dying Vaishnava. In general, hospice nurses do not spend a lengthy time at the home, but will make a few home visits every week, depending on the need. Their job is to assess the patient for pain and other symptom management as well as to make themselves available for emotional support for the patient, family, and other caregivers, if desired. An experienced hospice nurse will take the time to answer questions from the patient and caregivers. Not all nurses can care for the dying, and a good hospice nurse can offer many valuable services. Presently, our ISKCON movement has a few trained nurses in this field, but our hope is to increase this number through awareness of its need, as well as its many transcendental rewards.

Whether you are caring for a family member, senior Vaishnava, godbrother, or godsister, you have a challenging time ahead of you. This book is meant to serve as a guide so the reader may understand the hospice philosophy and how it relates to Krishna consciousness, basic terminology and concepts, and care of the patient from a Vaishnava perspective. I humbly offer this book as a service to my spiritual master, His Divine Grace A.C. Bhaktivedanta Swami Prabhupada, as well as to all the Vaishnava devotees of this world who are serving Lord Chaitanya's movement by caring for each other.

Sangita Devi Dasi
Krishna-Balaram Mandir
Vrindavan, India
March 21, 2000

Revised Edition
December 16, 2010
Moksada Ekadasi, Gita Jayanti

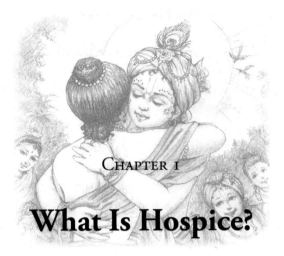

Chapter 1

What Is Hospice?

A History of the Hospice Movement

In medieval times, weary travelers on their way to or from the holy land on religious pilgrimage found rest, food, and comfort at monasteries along the way. Because the journey was often long and harsh, many travelers became ill and spent their final days at these shelters, which were eventually known as hospices. The word "hospice" is derived from the Latin word "*hospitium*," meaning a guesthouse. At these safe havens, under the care of benevolent strangers, many of them monks and nuns, these weak and dying pilgrims found refuge. Much later, in 1879, the Irish Sisters of Charity opened hospices in Dublin, and then in London in 1905. They believed that death was one stage of a longer journey.

Over time, this concept was all but lost until a reawakening occurred in the 1960s when Dr. Cicely Saunders, a British physician, founded the modern hospice movement. At St. Christopher's Hospice near London, Dr. Saunders developed a model for hospice care. She is credited with starting the first program to use modern pain management for compassionate care of the dying. She also taught that the dying patient and family should be treated holistically, caring for their emotional, mental, and spiritual needs. Dr. Saunders' contributions to the modern hospice movement cannot be compared.

In the United States, the National Hospice Organization was formed in 1979. In 1983, Congress passed the Medicare Hospice Benefit. It was not until 1988 that the International Hospice Institute helped form the Academy of Hospice Physicians.

At present, there are thousands of hospice programs in the United

States alone. Some provide an inpatient unit, usually in a wing of a hospital or in a long-term care facility which offers symptom management in acute situations, short-term respite for the caregivers when needed, and 24-hour nursing care when home care is not possible.

But, hospice is not a place. Most hospice care occurs in the home. It is an ideal achieved through a team approach for the care and comfort of the dying patient. Generally, this team consists of a physician who is knowledgeable in pain and other symptom management, a hospice nurse trained in holistic care, a nurse's aide who assists with bathing, skin care and other comfort measures, a pastor or other spiritual counselor, a social worker, a bereavement counselor, and volunteers who visit the patient in the home. The caregiver, who is usually a family member or close friend, is an integral part of the team. The professional members of the team educate, encourage, and support the patient, family members, and caregivers. Each member of the team should complement the other. Together, they assist in improving the final days of the patient and provide emotional and spiritual support for his or her loved ones.

In a sense, the International Society for Krishna Consciousness (ISKCON) presently stands on the brink of expanding the hospice movement by integrating the knowledge of hospice care for the dying with the spiritual wisdom given to us by Srila Prabhupada. Increasingly, we hear about devotees in our movement requiring end-of-life care. We need to embrace this situation as an ever-expanding opportunity to serve the Vaishnavas. If we gather our spiritual strength by taking shelter of Srila Prabhupada's teachings and also learning the concepts and practicalities of hospice care, we can, as a movement, develop a Krishna-conscious hospice program to care for those devotees in need of such a service.

In the *Bhagavad-gita As It Is* (2.27), Lord Krishna tells Arjuna, "For one who has taken birth, death is certain; and for one who is dead, birth is certain."

Who among us will not be in need of this service at some point in our own lives? If we rise to this challenge, surely His Divine Grace will be pleased.

Hospice and Palliative Care

According to the World Health Organization, palliative care is "the active total care of patients whose disease is not responsive to curative treatment. Control of pain, of other symptoms, and of psychological, social, and spiritual problems is paramount. The goal of palliative care is achievement of the best possible quality of life for patients and their families... Palliative care has its origin in the hospice movement."

The two terms, hospice care and palliative care, refer to the holistic care of the patient. Both provide pain and symptom management. Palliative treatments often involve surgery, radiation therapy, and chemotherapy, for example, as a means for pain and symptom control. These same treatments can also be performed as aggressive treatments in hopes of "curing" the disease. In hospice care, however, a cure is not considered possible and there is no longer hope of prolonging life. The goal of hospice and palliative care is to give the patient the best possible quality of remaining life. Generally, a patient should be encouraged to accept hospice care when his or her prognosis is six months or less. This allows time for emotional and spiritual counseling so the patient and family members can accept the inevitable. For a devotee, this process does not differ.

Hospice care encompasses a philosophy that embraces six concepts:

- Death is a natural part of life. When death is inevitable, hospice will neither seek to hasten nor postpone it.

- The clinical goal of hospice is to establish pain and other symptom management.

- Hospice recognizes death as a spiritual and physical experience. Psychological and spiritual pain are as significant as physical pain.

- The patient, family and loved ones are cared for as one unit.

- Hospice care includes bereavement counseling for loved ones after the death of the patient.

- Hospice care should be made available to patients and families in need regardless of their ability to pay.

A patient receiving hospice care is often referred for palliative treatments to relieve symptoms. Radiation therapy, for example, is often used to diminish the size of a tumor, thus reducing pain. In fact, palliative radiotherapy is the treatment of choice for cancer-related bone pain. This often improves the quality of life for the hospice patient. When considering these options, it is important for the patient to make an educated decision, weighing the side effects of such treatments against the pain or other symptoms he or she is experiencing.

For example, I spent one year caring for my husband's mother who was dying of breast cancer that had metastasized (spread) to the liver, lymphatic system, bone, and lungs. Although she was receiving hospice care, the pain in her pelvic area caused by a tumor was preventing her from walking. After discussing with her the possible side effects of radiation therapy, such as skin redness, burning, nausea, and vomiting, she decided to proceed with palliative radiation. After only a few weeks, her pain was significantly reduced and she was able to walk with a cane for a few months longer. Side effects were few and the radiation therapy improved the quality of her remaining life.

On the contrary, I also cared for a hospice patient whose physician had recommended simultaneous chemotherapy and radiation treatments to reduce a tumor in his lung. If successful, his breathing would have become less labored. Instead, uncontrollable side effects such as a sore throat, nausea, vomiting, skin burns, and fatigue made his daily life unbearable. After fully understanding that his lung cancer would quickly spread if these palliative treatments were stopped, this man chose to live out the remainder of his life using less aggressive symptom management techniques. Being allowed to make a well-informed decision about treatment options allowed him some minute control at a time when he was discovering just how powerless he really was.

Experiencing a Terminal Illness

As devotees of Lord Krishna, we practice *bhakti-yoga* as a means for self-realization. We try to live each day, each moment, serving Lord Krishna and our *guru*. We are intellectually aware that death can come at any moment, but even the great Vaishnava Yudhisthir Maharaj observed that the greatest wonder in this world is that we see living beings die all around us, yet we still believe that this will never happen to us. This form of denial is the greatest illusion in the material world.

When a devotee is diagnosed with a terminal illness it is quite sobering, to say the least. Suddenly he must confront what he has always accepted intellectually, that death can come at any moment. Yet, because each of us stands in a different place on the spiritual path of Krishna consciousness, we will all feel differently receiving such a prognosis. Of course, we all know that the ultimate goal of life is to become pure in our Krishna consciousness. We can remind the dying devotee that it is the greatest blessing to know when we are going to die. Realistically, though, not every devotee will remember this after being told he has six months or less to live.

Each of us brings into the illness our own fears, needs, past experiences, and conditioning. Therefore, it is important to be sensitive to the mental, emotional, and spiritual pain the dying devotee may experience.

Devotees, regardless of ashram, must be allowed the freedom to express their feelings and emotions concerning their impending death. Without these anxieties being addressed, a devotee will not become peaceful. Without peace, how can he remember Krishna?

The following are some expected–and perhaps some unexpected–emotional anxieties that the devotee may experience. The caregiver's role is to empathize with the devotee, to reassure him, and to be a "sounding board" when needed. At times, the patience of the caregiver may be tested. Please note that not everyone will experience these thoughts and emotions. They are simply common anxieties observed in many patients:

- Loss of control. Major and daily decisions that impact my life appear to be taken from me.

- Uncomfortable. Visitors tend to have superficial conversations and avoid eye contact due to their own discomfort. They seem horrified at seeing the physical changes caused by my disease.

- Deprived of my individuality. I am not given the freedom to express my feelings and emotions for fear of being criticized or even laughed at.

- Vulnerable. I find myself experiencing mood swings, sometimes within the same day or hour. Sometimes I want to be alone and sometimes I want the comfort of others.

- Fear. Even though I have firm faith in my spiritual beliefs, I sometimes experience momentary doubts. I am afraid to express this to anyone. This makes me afraid to die. I am also afraid of the pain I am facing with this disease.

- Anger. I find myself asking, "Why?" I wanted to do so much more in my life. What will happen to my family? I sometimes get angry with the Lord for doing this to me.

- Guilt. I feel guilty for having these fears and anger. I should be stronger. I feel like a burden to my caregivers.

- Sad. I feel alone. No one can relate to what I'm going through.

Making the Decision

When a devotee is given a prognosis of six months or less, important decisions must be made concerning care. Perhaps the devotee has been receiving aggressive treatment for his illness, such as chemotherapy or radiation therapy, as a means to heal the disease. If so, doctors should now be advising him that it is futile to continue with such treatments as a cure because the illness has progressed to the point of being incurable. Comfort care, rather than cure, is now in order.

In a study reported in the February 19, 2000 issue of the *British Medical Journal*, it was found that physicians are often too optimistic in their prognoses. On average, doctors predicted that their dying patients would live five times longer than they actually did. Obviously, this adversely affected the medical, financial, and social decisions made by the dying patients and their families. Often patients are encouraged to continue seeking aggressive, though ineffective, treatments, which delay palliative care for comfort.

Not all healthcare professionals agree with this approach. For example, in the April 24, 2000 issue of *Advance for Nurses*, Terri Maxwell, MSN, RN, AOCN, and executive director for the Center for Palliative Care, states, "Physicians generally are so disease-oriented that they often keep walking down the road of more treatment. At times, patients are offered more treatment because it is easier than having honest conversations about end-of-life care." She further explains, "If you keep offering treatments, some (patients) will want that treatment. We should help them realize that when a cure is no longer possible, there are a great deal of things that can be done to make them comfortable."

Although the latter approach is often more realistic, it has been my experience that some doctors, even oncologists who specialize in treating cancer patients, will hesitate to be direct with a patient when cure is no longer an option. I have heard doctors tell patients, "We are going to treat the symptoms now rather than the disease."

To the non-medical patient this can be confusing and misleading. Similarly, other medical personnel, including nurses, are often equally uncomfortable with the direct approach when speaking with a patient who is hospice-appropriate. If you are hearing an "indirect approach" from the physician, you have the right to ask questions. Below are some suggestions:

- What is the prognosis?

- Should we consider any aggressive treatments, such as surgery, radiation therapy, or chemotherapy? Is it too late for such measures as a cure?

- Would these or other treatments be helpful in prolonging my life?

- Would these or other treatments, when used as palliative measures, help ease the pain?

- Would you recommend hospice care at this time?

And remember, you always have the right to a second—and even third—opinion from another physician!

Once the devotee makes the decision to accept hospice care, his work is just beginning. He will experience a physical, emotional, mental, and spiritual transformation. I have told many patients and families who are new to hospice that there is such a thing as a "good death." As devotees, we know this to be true. If someone is physically, emotionally, and mentally pain-free, has other symptoms managed well, and is rightly situated spiritually, he will experience an auspicious, most glorious passing away.

Your role as a caregiver, combined with strong support from the devotee community, can help achieve this for the dying devotee.

Spiritual Care in Hospice

In many ways, the hospice philosophy of caring for the spiritual needs of the patient coincide with our Krishna consciousness philosophy. In both, death is a natural occurrence to be eventually experienced by everyone. Both teach that spiritual distress is universal in those confronting imminent death. Both encourage spiritual support. It would be difficult, however, to find two hospice professionals (even clergy) to agree on the meaning of "spiritual care."

When one is dying of a terminal illness, spiritual issues have a way of surfacing and moving to the forefront. It is easy for a medical professional (even one working in a hospice) to miss or ignore spiritual pain. In his book, *Notes on Symptom Control in Hospice and Palliative Care*, Dr. Peter Kaye writes about the patient who may say, "I seem to be wasting away," or "I'm not eating enough." Kaye states, "It is tempting for the doctor to respond by asking about diet or dysphagia (difficulty swallowing) when it is fear of not existing that the patient is struggling to express."

Most hospice patients I have cared for expressed the importance of a strong spiritual faith when facing death. I encouraged them all to become more introspective at a very crucial time in their lives. Whether they were Catholic, Protestant, Jewish, or Buddhist, I held their hands and prayed with them. With some, we discussed the meaning of life as they saw it. Many wished to talk about heaven and hell. Some even mentioned reincarnation as a "possibility." I gave them all *prasadam*, gave them flowers that had been offered to Krishna, and even had some taste *caranamrta* from the Deities. I never told them to believe in something different from what they had trusted to be true their entire lives. I simply helped them to get in touch with their beliefs even more. It is interesting to note that I have cared for only one patient who professed to be an "atheist." From the time he entered the inpatient hospice unit he remained depressed in spite of receiving antidepressant medications and a great deal of emotional support from the staff. He refused visits from the pastor and spoke often about there being "nothing after death." Unfortunately, this poor man died very angry.

As a caregiver for a devotee you carry a big advantage. You both share the same beliefs and maintain the same goal of life. And what is that goal?

In the *Bhagavad-gita* (2.51), Lord Krishna instructs Arjuna, "The wise, engaged in devotional service, take refuge in the Lord, and free themselves from the cycle of birth and death by renouncing the fruits of action in the material world. In this way they can attain that state beyond all miseries."

It is natural for devotees to speak about spiritual topics because it is a part of the Krishna-conscious process for self-realization. In general, devotees are very comfortable discussing death and dying. If you are fortunate enough to also have a support group of devotees in your community then you, the caregiver, as well as the devotee you are caring for, can take shelter in the soothing comfort of that association. But "spiritual topics" often exclude discussing "spiritual pain," which for the dying devotee may take many forms, including fear, doubts, and a sense of urgency to become more spiritually enlightened. A good caregiver should not only be a good advisor, but a good listener and friend as well.

Srila Prabhupada writes in the *Bhagavad-gita* (6.32): "One who is Krishna conscious is a *yogi*; he is aware of everyone's happiness and distress by dint of his own personal experience. The cause of the distress of a living entity is forgetfulness of his relationship with God. And the cause of happiness is knowing Krishna to be the supreme enjoyer of all the activities of the human being… A devotee of the Lord always looks to the welfare of all living entities, and in this way he is factually a friend of everyone."

The Dying Devotee's Bill of Rights

Once someone chooses to accept hospice care, he should be aware of some basic rights to which he is entitled. They are as follows:

- I have the right to participate in decisions concerning my care.

- I have the right to expect continuing medical attention even though my illness is incurable.

- I have the right to be free from pain.

- I have the right to have my questions answered honestly.

- I have the right not to be deceived.

- I have the right to express my feelings and emotions about my approaching death.

- I have the right to discuss and expand my spiritual realizations during this dying process.

- I have the right to die in the Krishna conscious environment I choose.

- I have the right to die with dignity.

- I have the right to expect my wishes to be respected regarding what will happen to my body after death.

- I have the right to have help for my family in accepting my death.

- I have the right to be cared for by caring, sensitive, knowledgeable people who will attempt to understand my needs and gain satisfaction in helping me face my death.

Any lesser treatment of the dying Vaishnava would be an enormous injustice.

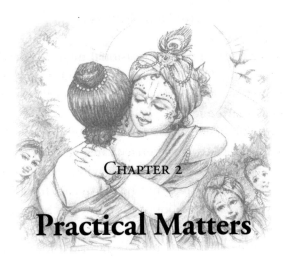

Chapter 2

Practical Matters

Who will Care for the Vaishnava?

When a devotee is diagnosed with a terminal illness, one of the first things to consider is who will care for the patient. The desires of the dying devotee are of the utmost importance and should always be considered first when making such a decision. If you are the wife, husband, or adult child you may want to be the primary caregiver. The primary caregiver coordinates and is responsible for the majority of care. Of course, the primary caregiver cannot expect to care for the patient alone. When first diagnosed, a hospice patient may not require round-the-clock care. He may be able to do some things by himself, such as bathing, dressing, and preparing meals. This independence should be encouraged. But as his condition declines he will require more and more care from others. Although you may want to, it is not humanly possible for one person to perform 24-hour care. That is why a team of caregivers, even if that means one or two people who can relieve you, should be considered.

Naturally, the *ashram* of the devotee must be taken into consideration. If the devotee requiring care is a *brahmacari* or *sannyasi*, then obviously a male caregiver should administer personal care. Similarly, if the devotee needing care is an unmarried lady, a female caregiver is in order.

If you wish to be a caregiver, certain factors must be measured. Are you healthy enough to perform care that most likely will involve physical strain? Often a hospice patient requires lifting, turning, repositioning, and assistance with walking. Even if the patient does not require this when first diagnosed, it is inevitable that he will. Depending on the size and weight of the patient, this can be very strenuous on the caregiver's back, neck and limbs.

Being a caregiver often means occasional nights of sleep deprivation. This can be exhausting. Can someone relieve you during the day so you can rest? If you are not refreshed you will not be much help to your patient, who needs you at your best.

Do you have a job in which you can take a temporary leave of absence? Being a caregiver, especially the primary caregiver, can be a full-time job in itself. If your income is required, then leaving your job to take on such a tremendous responsibility may not be financially feasible. In that case, alternate caregivers who are willing to care for the patient when you are working may be the answer.

When my mother-in-law became ill she asked me to be her primary caregiver. But she also had nine adult children. When she eventually required 24-hour care, I called a family meeting. I presented a copy of their mother's living will and discussed her wishes to receive comfort care only. I taught them about her medication schedule, how to evaluate her pain level, when and how to give additional medications for symptom management, the use of an oxygen tank, and how to give a bed bath. I also had a sign-up sheet for three 8-hour shifts per day. We made a month-long schedule on a calendar that hung in the kitchen.

My home phone number, work number, and cellular phone number were posted in clear sight for emergencies. We also listed the home phone number, work number, and beeper number of each caregiver. Then we devised a "phone tree" in which one caregiver would call the next one in line, and so forth, in case of a change in their mother's condition. This way, no one person was responsible to call everyone. I also hung a large sign that read "DO NOT CALL 911" to remind everyone that my mother-in-law had advance directives in her living will that specifically stated that she did not want heroic measures performed on her, such as cardiopulmonary resuscitation (CPR) when her heartbeat and respirations ceased. If one of her caregivers had panicked and called the paramedics to her home when one of those events had occurred, it would have infringed upon her basic rights as a hospice patient.

To increase communication, when one caregiver came on his or her shift, the previous caregiver gave a "nursing report." We also kept a notepad next to each medication bottle and recorded when each one was due and the times when additional medications for symptom management were administered. Memory is short in this Age of Kali and accurate notes are essential. I remained the primary caregiver, but organizing a "caregiver team" to relieve one another every eight hours avoided caregiver "burnout." (This subject will be discussed in detail in Chapter 9.)

The following are some topics that can be included in your own report to fellow caregivers:

- What routine medications were given on your shift?

- Did the patient complain of increased pain? What additional medications were given to relieve the pain? Did it work?

- Did the patient exhibit shortness of breath or anxiety, and what medications were given for symptom management? What time were they given? What was the outcome of these interventions? (Remember to write the time these medications were given on the notepad next to the prescription bottle.)

- Did the patient experience any gastrointestinal problems such as constipation, diarrhea, or nausea? What was done to alleviate the discomfort? How often did he use the bathroom or bedpan? Was he continent?

- What and how much did the patient eat during your shift?

- Did the patient sleep? How long?

- Was the patient bathed or massaged during your shift?

- Were the patient's teeth brushed? Mouth refreshed?

- What skin care was performed, such as the application of lotion or repositioning to avoid bedsores?

- Did the patient discuss his or her impending death?

- Did the patient verbalize any spiritual anxiety concerning his or her situation?

- What is the patient's level of consciousness at present—very alert, slightly confused, incoherent, or unresponsive?

This report can be modified according to your particular situation. It is important to remember that accurate recording of medication administration and other interventions, as well as close verbal communication, are the keys to a successful caregiver team.

The chart at the end of the chapter, created by Jusaniya Dasi (Judy Harris, RNC, BSN, CHPN), a disciple of Srila Prabhupada and a long-time nurse, can be enlarged and copied as it appears or used as an example and modified in order to increase communication between caregivers. Using a chart such as this one is optional, but since many changes can occur within one day in a dying patient, it is beneficial to keep an accurate written record.

Where will the Vaishnava be Cared for?

Whether a devotee is living in a temple building or will be cared for at home, many things must be considered in order to render the best possible care. This list will need to be adjusted according to the medical condition of the patient at the time of diagnosis. Additional considerations will have to be examined as the patient's condition deteriorates.

If the devotee resides in a temple, please consider the following:

- Does the devotee have a private room? Does he have a private bathroom, close to the bedroom? (A private room is a necessity. It would be very helpful if the patient had a private bathroom, but this may not always be possible.)

- Is the devotee's room situated in a quiet area of the temple so rest will not be disturbed?

- Does the room have air conditioning or fans for summer months, an adequate heating system for winter months, proper ventilation (preferably two windows with screens for a slight cross breeze in the spring and fall), and proper lighting fixtures that provide both a bright light and dim lighting when needed? (Even the number of electrical outlets in the room needs to be considered. Often a great deal of medical equipment is required, such as an oxygen concentrator or a humidifier. Care must be taken to avoid electrical overload that can be a fire hazard.)

- What type of bed is required? Traditional bedding on the floor is not always practical for a devotee patient. The floor may be drafty, for instance, which may cause the devotee to needlessly suffer with chills. Also, noise from the room below can be disturbing when sleeping low to the floor. Depending on his medical condition, the devotee may require softer bedding. Again, consider the desires of the ill devotee, but encourage what is practical according to his particular situation. Would the devotee be more comfortable on a bed with a mattress, box spring, and frame? Does he require side-rails on one or both sides for safety? (Several situations may warrant the use of a hospital bed with side-rails, such as confusion, hallucinations, unsteady gait when standing alone, and previous falls when attempting to get out of bed without assistance. A hospital bed with adjustable head and foot controls may be useful for comfort even if side-rails are not required.) Would a hospital bed fit in the room? How difficult would it be to have a hospital bed delivered if the devotee's room is situated on a top floor of a temple? (Most medical equipment companies that rent hospital beds try very hard to accommodate special needs.)

- Is the devotee able to walk unassisted? Does he require one-person assistance? Two-person assistance? Does he live in a room that requires walking up and down stairs to gain access? If so, does the temple have a room on the ground floor that can be used? (Even if the devotee is able to climb stairs at the beginning of his diagnosis, most likely this will become increasingly difficult and eventually impossible. It would be easier for all concerned if a move was made to a ground-floor room before the devotee becomes weak and nonambulatory.) Does the devotee require a wheelchair? Is the temple wheelchair-accessible with ramps?

- Is there a kitchen available to prepare special *prasadam* for the devotee, if needed? Is there a refrigerator close by to keep bottled water, juices, and medications that require refrigeration?

- Where will the caregivers stay? Can they stay close enough so the ill devotee can be heard and have his needs met day or night? (It is a good idea to provide the devotee with a bell to ring when needing assistance. Ideally, one caregiver should be within hearing range at all times. Room monitors used for babies are useful, but do not always clearly transmit. Also, frequent battery checks are required.)

- Is the room large enough to accommodate visitors if desired by the devotee?

- Can the devotee be easily transported to the temple room to have *darshan* of the Deities?

If the devotee will be cared for in a private home, then obviously not all of the above will need to be considered. Still, the following should be well thought out:

- Will the devotee be cared for in a ground-floor apartment or a one-story home so transport, if needed, is more feasible? If the devotee lives in a two-story home, should she be cared for in a downstairs bedroom, if available, or in a living room, for example, where she can be observed and heard more easily? (Some patients prefer this to the seclusion of an upstairs bedroom.)

- If it is decided that the devotee will be cared for downstairs, is there a way to screen or curtain off a section of the room for the patient's privacy?

- Is there a bathroom downstairs? Will a bedside commode be needed? (Again, the privacy issue must be considered.)

- Is the home wheelchair-accessible?

- Is the home in a quiet neighborhood? Is one room quieter than another?

- Does one room get more sunlight than another?

- Does the room have air conditioning, fans, good lighting, and adequate circulation? Will a portable heater be necessary if the room is drafty?

- Does the devotee require a special bed such as a hospital bed? Where will it best fit?

- Can the devotee see the household Deities from where she is resting? Are there pictures of Krishna in his room? Can they be seen from where he is positioned? Is there a sound system so he can listen to recordings of *bhajans* and lectures?

- If desired, how can the devotee be transported to the nearest temple to have *darshan* of the Deities and have association with other devotees? Would he be driven in a car? Can he be taken in a wheelchair?

- Are there devotees in your community who can visit the home and read Srila Prabhupada's books to the devotee?

- Are there devotees in your community who can occasionally provide *prasadam* for the patient and caregivers? Go grocery shopping? Assist with laundry?

Each situation requires individual consideration. In a hospice situation, plans cannot be "carved in stone" because circumstances rapidly change—sometimes on a daily basis. Creativity and flexibility are required to adjust to an ever-changing situation. However, if you begin the care with a well-thought-out plan, keeping in mind that adjustments will need to be made as events are altered, you will avoid unnecessary frustration and anxiety in the future.

Should we Travel to the Holy Dhama?

In the *Bhagavad-gita* (8.21) Srila Prabhupada writes in his purport, "Krishna's supreme abode and Krishna Himself are nondifferent, being of the same quality. On this earth, Vrindavan, ninety miles southeast of Delhi, is a replica of that supreme Goloka Vrindavan located in the spiritual sky. When Krishna descended on this earth, He sported on that particular tract of land known as Vrindavan in the district of Mathura, India."

Being able to leave one's body in the place where Lord Krishna performed His transcendental pastimes is a most auspicious event. Such a fortunate soul as this would surely receive the Lord's blessings. But such a situation must be well planned, since living in the holy *dhama* means added austerities. Even the lengthy plane ride is rigorous and must be realistically decided upon according to the medical needs and physical strength of the dying devotee. Being accompanied by a caregiver who can administer medications, provide *prasadam*, and manipulate any special equipment (such as portable oxygen tank, if needed) is essential.

Since the first edition of this book was published, His Holiness Giriraj Swami has overseen the construction of a well-equipped and beautiful hospice facility in the holy *dhama* of Vrindavan, India, called the Bhaktivedanta Hospice. This inpatient hospice has its own temple room with Jagannatha Deities and is also just a few-minute walk from the Krishna-Balaram Mandir. However, if your patient prefers to stay elsewhere in India, you need to consider the following factors. To begin, one would need to arrange for adequate housing. Ideally, it should be clean and comfortable, have a generator for electrical backup due to frequent power outages, have proper lighting and circulation, air conditioning and/or fans for the hot summer months, some type of heating system for the winter months, have cooking facilities with a refrigerator, and a private "western-style" bathroom. It would be best if the room were on the ground floor and was wheelchair-accessible.

It should be noted that many drugs routinely used in hospice and palliative care in the West are either difficult to get or unavailable in India. In addition, some of India's pharmaceutical companies produce medicine in compound formulas, so the devotee may be taking unnecessary medications along with the ones that are needed. Medicines in India often come in injectable or tablet form only. As of this writing, alternate routes to oral medications such as rectal or sublingual (medications that dissolve under the tongue) are fairly new concepts in some places in India. Medications given by intramuscular (IM) injection are rarely used in hospice care. For a hospice patient who is eating poorly and who may even be emaciated, IM injections can be uncomfortable and unnecessary. Suppository medications and/or concentrated liquid pain medicines given under the tongue are often required if a hospice patient is eventually unable to swallow tablets.

Further, in smaller villages it may be difficult to find a qualified medical physician. Some who are pharmacists refer to themselves as doctors. At available medical facilities, cleanliness and safe practices are often substandard. I personally found the conditions in one village hospital to be shocking. When I expressed concern to a physician at this hospital, he said, "This is India. It is dirty out there and it is dirty in here!"

In the holy *dhama* of Vrindavan, however, modern medical facilities are beginning to open. Care for the terminally ill is also improving, most notably with the establishment of the Bhaktivedanta Hospice, inspired and guided by His Holiness Giriraj Swami and staffed by Vaishnava physicians and nurses.

Even with the added austerities of traveling to and staying in India, the spiritual benefits of leaving one's body in the holy land where Lord Krishna once walked are beyond compare. With proper arrangements, it can be the most auspicious situation for a Vaishnava whose death is imminent.

Choosing a Hospice in the West

If it is decided that a devotee will remain in the West, then finding a local hospice to assist you is sensible. A good hospice agency can arrange for special medical equipment, including a hospital bed, begin the devotee on a medication regime for pain and other symptom management, provide nursing visits and continual assessments, arrange for a nursing assistant to provide personal care, if desired, and provide a social worker and bereavement counselor to assist the patient as well as the family. Every hospice agency employs a physician as its medical director who is on call for medication orders, emergencies, etc. A patient has the right to continue seeing his or her primary physician or specialist, or to become a full-time patient of the hospice physician.

Finding a local hospice agency that will come to your home or temple is not difficult. The following list should help you begin:

1) Ask the physician who has given a prognosis of six months or less and has recommended hospice care. Most likely he or she works with one or two hospice agencies and can refer you to one.

2) If the devotee has been in the hospital, ask the hospital discharge planner to recommend a local hospice agency.

3) If the devotee has private medical insurance, call the customer service number and ask if they can assist you in locating a nearby agency.

4) Check your local yellow pages under "Hospice." (Many hospitals have their own home hospice agency.)

5) Call or visit the website of the American Cancer Society for information and referrals.

6) Call your state's Department of Social Services and ask for assistance.

Below is a list of some hospice organizations that may be helpful. Each one offers a variety of information. I have noted the organizations that will assist you in finding a local hospice.

- **Vaisnavas C.A.R.E.**
  Website: www.vaisnavascare.org

Vaisnavas C.A.R.E. (Counseling, Assistance, Resource, and Education) is a worldwide network of volunteers who offer their support to the terminally ill and their loved ones. Through education, website support, and volunteer assistance, Vaisnavas C.A.R.E. (aka V-C.A.R.E.) offers comfort to those in need by integrating the knowledge of caring for the terminally ill with the spiritual wisdom given by His Divine Grace A.C. Bhaktivedanta Swami Prabhupada. An online course is included at no charge on this website that can give one a basic understanding of caring for the terminally ill.

- **Final Journey Seminars**
  Website: www.finaljourneyseminars.com

This organization offers a free seminar for the Hindu community about end of life medical choices, religious services, cremation, legal issues, and financial planning.

- **Hospice Link**
  Website: www.hospiceworld.org

Telephone: 207-255-8800

This is a telephone service offered by the Hospice Education Institute in Maine. They provide referrals to local hospice agencies throughout the United States. They are an excellent source for information on hospice and palliative care—not only for nonmedical persons, but for healthcare professionals as well.

- **Help the Hospices**
  Website: www.helpthehospices.org.uk

This is the leading charity supporting hospice care throughout the UK. If you are a patient, caregiver, or have an interest in hospice and palliative care, explore this site for information, support or to get involved.

- **Hospice Foundation of America**
  1710 Rhode Island Avenue, NW
  Suite 400
  Washington, DC 20036
  Website: www.hospicefoundation.org
  Toll-free number: 800-854-3402

Among other subjects, this website has a wealth of information on grieving for a loved one who has passed away.

- **International Association for Hospice and Palliative Care**
  Website: www.hospicecare.com

This non-profit organization is dedicated to promoting hospice and palliative care worldwide.

- **CancerNet**
  Website: www.cancernet.nci.nih.gov

This website provides recent information from the National Cancer Institute. Some topics include: Types of Cancer, Treatment Options, Support and Resources, and Clinical Trial Results.

- **Children's Hospice International (CHI)**
  1101 King Street
  Suite 360
  Alexandria, VA 22314 U.S.A.
  Website: www.chionline.org/

This site gives valuable information on pediatric hospice services. CHI provides education, training, and technical assistance to those who care for children with life-threatening conditions and their families.

- **The National Family Caregivers Association**
  Website: www.nfcacares.org

This site provides education and information to caregivers, including state and federal agencies in the United States, intended to improve the quality of life of those who are caring for an ill, elderly, or disabled person. The Association has many resources listed, as well as a page for you to connect with other caregivers.

- **American Pain Foundation**
  Website: www.painfoundation.org

This is an independent nonprofit organization whose mission is to improve the quality of life of people with pain by raising public awareness, providing practical information, and advocating to remove barriers and raise awareness of effective pain management.

- **Dying Well**
  Website: www.dyingwell.org

This site is a helpful resource for people facing life-limiting illness, their families, and their professional caregivers.

- **Children's Hospice and Palliative Care Coalition**
  Website: www.childrenshospice.org

This is a social movement led by children's hospitals, hospices, home health agencies, and individuals to improve care for children with life-threatening conditions and their families.

- **Growth House, Inc.**
  Website: www.growthhouse.org

This website provides links to resources for life-threatening illness and end-of-life care. Their mission is to improve the quality of compassionate care for people who are dying through education and global professional collaboration. This site gives you access to a comprehensive collection of reviewed resources for end-of-life care.

Once you have contacted a hospice agency, you may want to first inquire about available services and financial arrangements. They should be able to tell you if they provide resources that can find financial assistance for the patient, if needed.

Very often, the hospice social worker can enlist whatever community assistance is available. (All hospice agencies have their own funding for a limited amount of patients who are unable to pay and do not have medical insurance. Some also offer payment plan options.) Hospice services are covered under Medicare Part A, and currently 46 states in the U.S. finance hospice care for those who qualify under their Medicaid program. In addition, hospice care is a covered benefit under most private insurance plans, HMOs, and other managed care organizations. If the patient does not have medical insurance or a prescription payment plan, then the hospice staff should be able to tell you which pharmacies in your city have more affordable rates for prescription medications. Also, medications ordered by generic names are less expensive than those ordered by the trade name. (For example, acetaminophen is the generic name for Tylenol, which is the trade name.)

Hospice agencies may advertise themselves as "Medicare certified" and/or "JCAHO certified." Simply stated, Medicare certification means they have met federal minimum requirements for care and management. JCAHO stands for the Joint Commission on Accreditation of Healthcare Organizations, which is a nationally-recognized accrediting institute. If the hospice agency has sought and received accreditation, it is committed to providing the highest standard of patient and family care. It is a good idea to question the hospice agency about certification and accreditation.

The following are other questions you may want to ask:

- Does the agency have a nurse on call 24 hours a day? Will he or she make a visit to the home in the middle of the night in an emergency situation?

- How often will the primary nurse visit the home per week? What will he or she do during these visits? Who will visit on his or her day off? Will the alternate nurse be familiar with the patient's medical condition? What does a nursing assistant do? If desired, how often will he or she visit?

- Who does the "care team" consist of? (Social worker? Counselor?)

- Who is the Medical Director of the agency? Will he or she work closely with the patient's own physician?

- What assistance is available for family members, such as bereavement counseling?

- Does the agency provide medications? Does it provide necessary medical equipment?

- Does the agency provide inpatient care in a hospice unit, hospital, or long-term care facility? Would this option be available for crisis situations? Would it be available to the patient as a way to provide respite for the caregivers?

It is important that the patient and caregivers feel comfortable with the hospice nurse who will first come to the home or temple to make an initial assessment. He or she will evaluate the patient to see if he meets the hospice criteria. The patient, caregivers, and family members need to feel satisfied with the nurse's answers to their questions. This might also be a good time to mention the devotee's vegetarian diet so the nurse is aware of what can and cannot be recommended for nutrition. (A good nurse will be nonjudgemental and may even welcome a new opportunity to care for a devotee of Lord Krishna. Many hospice nurses enjoy learning about cultural and religious differences from their patients and families.)

Living Wills

During the initial visit, the hospice nurse will ask if the patient has a living will. If not, he or she can usually provide you with one to sign. The purpose of a living will is to have a written record of the patient's wishes concerning treatment that will unnecessarily prolong life. It is a legal document that is signed, dated, and witnessed, and serves as an advance directive should the patient be unable to express her desires at the time such treatment might be administered. Some living wills state one's wishes only in the case of a terminal illness. Most likely, this will be the type available from the hospice agency. Other living wills state what a person would want done (or not done) if he were in a state of permanent unconsciousness, as in the case of a serious accident, for instance. Some give up to six case scenarios with treatment options to be accepted or refused in various circumstances.

A living will protects a patient's right to die with dignity. It ensures that treatment will be limited to comfort measures and pain management, including any discomfort that might occur as a result of withholding life-sustaining treatment. It usually includes a checklist of interventions such as the following:

- I do/do not want cardiac resuscitation (including CPR and/or chemical resuscitation).

- I do/do not want mechanical respiration (to be placed on a ventilator).

- I do/do not want tube feeding or any other artificial or invasive form of nutrition (food) or hydration (water).

- I do/do not want blood or blood products.

- I do/do not want kidney dialysis.

- I do/do not want antibiotics. (If desired, you have the right to state that you will accept antibiotics for comfort measures only, but not to needlessly extend life as in the case of taking antibiotics to cure pneumonia.)

- I do/do not want intravenous (IV) medications.

Every living will is written differently. However, most will include a space for the patient to designate a Medical Power of Attorney (POA). This should be a well-trusted associate or family member who can make medical treatment decisions for the patient if he should become incompetent or is in a state of unconsciousness. The POA will speak on the patient's behalf to refuse or accept life-sustaining treatments if the patient is incapable of making these decisions. It is suggested that an alternate POA be listed on the living will in case the first choice is unable or unwilling to make a decision.

Every state differs in its requirements, but it is necessary for the Power of Attorney and the alternate to be of legal age. The hospice agency will keep a copy of the living will on file. Usually the original legal document is kept with the patient or primary caregiver.

Most living wills also provide room for "additional comments." Specific requests by the devotee should be written here. For example, "I request my family, friends, and caregivers to provide continuous chanting of the Hare Krishna mantra if I become unconscious or am too weak to chant myself."

Below is a copy of a living will written by Kusha Devi Dasi, a senior disciple of Srila Prabhupada. It is a fine example of a living will written specifically for Vaishnavas. In the United States living wills are now recognized in all 50 states, but each state has individual requirements. Therefore, it is recommended to seek consultation with an attorney in the final preparations of such a legal document.

A Living Will

To My Family, My Physician, My Clergyman, My Lawyer:

If the time comes when I can no longer take part in decisions for my own future, let this statement stand as the testament of my wishes:

If there is no reasonable expectation of my recovery from physical or mental disability,

I, _____ (Full legal name here),

- Request that I be allowed to die and not be kept alive by artificial means or heroic measures, including cardiopulmonary resuscitation (CPR), mechanical respiration, artificial or invasive means of nutrition or hydration, administration of blood or blood products, and intravenous medications that will unnecessarily prolong my life.

- Death is as much a reality as birth, growth, maturity, and old age— it is the one certainty. I do not fear death as much as I fear the indignity of deterioration and hopeless pain.

- Do not put any product or food containing meat, fish, or eggs into my body. This is in accordance with my belief system. I wish to maintain this standard in sickness and in health.

- I ask that a recording of the chanting of the Holy Names of Lord Krishna, sung or spoken by my spiritual master, A.C. Bhaktivedanta Swami Prabhupada, be played close to my ears constantly (24 hours a day), or transcendental sound vibrations such as *Srimad-Bhagavatam* or Krishna *bhajans* be mercifully administered to me without cessation up to the moment of death.

- If it is at all possible to take me to the Holy *Dhama* of Vrindavan, India for my final days, this is most desired.

- As recommended in the Vedic scriptures, I request that my body be cremated after death and that the ashes be placed in the Yamuna River in India. (If desired, other arrangements or specific instructions for a funeral service can be written below.)

Signed: _____
Date: _____
Witnessed by: _____
Witnessed by: _____

Medical Power of Attorney

I, the undersigned, _____ (Full legal name here) on this _____ day of _____ in the year _____ being of sound mind, willfully and voluntarily appoint_____ (Full legal name here) to accept or refuse medical treatment on my behalf and in my interest if, due to a condition resulting from illness or injury, and in the judgement of the attending physician, I become incapable of making a decision to accept or refuse medical treatment, food, and liquid.

Signed:_____
Address: _____

As Medical Power of Attorney I understand that acceptance of this appointment means I have a duty to act in good faith and with due regard for the interest and benefit of the person appointing me.

Signed:_____
Date: _____

If for any reason the above-appointed Medical Power of Attorney is unable or unwilling to carry out this act of duty,

I appoint, _____ (Full legal name here) to act as Alternate Medical Power of Attorney with the same rights and duties as stated above.

Signed:_____
Address: _____
Date: _____

At any time, a patient has the right to revoke his decision to continue with hospice and palliative care. He may also revoke any decisions stated in the living will. The hospice agency and the attending physician must be made aware of this revocation as soon as possible.

Advance directives are not to be confused with euthanasia, which is when a patient requests medical intervention to hasten death. Certainly a patient has the right to refuse life-sustaining treatment, but the Krishna consciousness philosophy and laws of *karma* do not allow for assisted death. With compassionate hospice care, a patient can receive comfort measures for physical, mental, emotional, and spiritual pain. He is given control as to what treatment he wants to accept or refuse. Having someone assist a patient with his death is not an option offered in hospice care.

Having cared for hundreds of hospice patients, I have had only a few ask me to administer a lethal dose of narcotics. Of course, I refused. But when a patient asks to be killed, it should be seen as a sign of severe hopelessness that cannot be ignored. I immediately contacted all members of the hospice team and gave each of these patients even more attention and support. I found more time on my shift to sit with them, hold their hands, and encourage them to verbalize their feelings, fears, and anguish. I became a better listener. I especially encouraged them to reflect on their belief in God as the Supreme Friend and Controller. In retrospect, these interventions helped each of these patients to feel a little less lonely on a very difficult and solitary journey.

	7:00 AM	8:00 AM	9:00 AM	10:00 AM	11:00 AM	12:00 PM	1:00 PM	2:00 PM
Level of Consciousness (L.O.C)								
Sleep								
Respiration								
Pain								
Other Symptoms (ie. dizziness, dry mouth, etc)								
Medication 1								
Medication 2								
Medication 3								
Medication 4								
Medication 5								
Therapy 1 (ie. ice/heat pack, etc)								
Therapy 2 (ie. ice/heat pack, etc)								

Mouth Care								
Skin Care								
Bath								
G.I								
B.M								
Urine								
Continent								
Food								
Drink								
Concerns								

Bodily Locations	Pain	L.O.C	G.I	Respirations
LA - left arm	1 - slight pain	A - awake	N - nausea	L - labored
RA - right arm	10 - most severe pain	AL - alert	V - vomiting	S - shallow
LL - left leg	ever experienced	O - oriented to	C - constipation	W - wheezing
RL - right leg		1. self	D - diarrhea	G - gasping
H - head		2. surroundings		E - easy
CH - chest		3. time		
Abd - abdomen		R - responsive		
		NR - non-responsive		

	3:00 PM	4:00 PM	5:00 PM	6:00 PM	7:00 PM	8:00 PM	9:00 PM	10:00 PM
Level of Consciousness (L.O.C)								
Sleep								
Respiration								
Pain								
Other Symptoms (ie. dizziness, dry mouth, etc)								
Medication 1								
Medication 2								
Medication 3								
Medication 4								
Medication 5								
Therapy 1 (ie. ice/heat pack, etc)								
Therapy 2 (ie. ice/heat pack, etc)								

Mouth Care								
Skin Care								
Bath								
G.I								
B.M								
Urine								
Continent								
Food								
Drink								
Concerns								

Bodily Locations	Pain	L.O.C	G.I	Respirations
LA - left arm	1 - slight pain	A - awake	N - nausea	L - labored
RA - right arm	10 - most severe pain	AL - alert	V - vomiting	S - shallow
LL - left leg	ever experienced	O - oriented to	C - constipation	W - wheezing
RL - right leg		1. self	D - diarrhea	G - gasping
H - head		2. surroundings		E - easy
CH - chest		3. time		
Abd - abdomen		R - responsive		
		NR - non-responsive		

	11:00 PM	12:00 PM	1:00 AM	2:00 AM	3:00 AM	4:00 AM	5:00 AM	6:00 AM
Level of Consciousness (L.O.C)								
Sleep								
Respiration								
Pain								
Other Symptoms (ie. dizziness, dry mouth, etc)								
Medication 1								
Medication 2								
Medication 3								
Medication 4								
Medication 5								
Therapy 1 (ie. ice/heat pack, etc)								
Therapy 2 (ie. ice/heat pack, etc)								

Mouth Care							
Skin Care							
Bath							
G.I							
B.M							
Urine							
Continent							
Food							
Drink							
Concerns							

Bodily Locations

LA - left arm
RA - right arm
LL - left leg
RL - right leg
H - head
CH - chest
Abd - abdomen

Pain

1 - slight pain
10 - most severe pain ever experienced

L.O.C

A - awake
AL - alert
O - oriented to
1. self
2. surroundings
3. time
R - responsive
NR - non-responsive

G.I

N - nausea
V - vomiting
C - constipation
D - diarrhea

Respirations

L - labored
S - shallow
W - wheezing
G - gasping
E - easy

	7:00 AM	8:00 AM	9:00 AM	10:00 AM	11:00 AM	12:00 PM	1:00 PM	2:00 PM
Level of Consciousness (L.O.C)								
Sleep								
Respiration								
Pain								
Other Symptoms (ie. dizziness, dry mouth, etc)								
Medication 1								
Medication 2								
Medication 3								
Medication 4								
Medication 5								
Therapy 1 (ie. ice/heat pack, etc)								
Therapy 2 (ie. ice/heat pack, etc)								

Mouth Care							
Skin Care							
Bath							
G.I							
B.M							
Urine							
Continent							
Food							
Drink							
Concerns							

Bodily Locations	Pain	L.O.C	G.I	Respirations
LA - left arm	1 - slight pain	A - awake	N - nausea	L - labored
RA - right arm	10 - most severe pain	AL - alert	V - vomiting	S - shallow
LL - left leg	ever experienced	O - oriented to	C - constipation	W - wheezing
RL - right leg		1. self	D - diarrhea	G - gasping
H - head		2. surroundings		E - easy
CH - chest		3. time		
Abd - abdomen		R - responsive		
		NR - non-responsive		

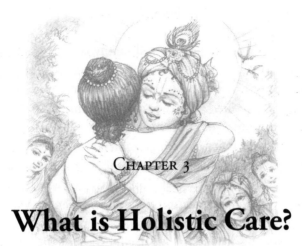

Chapter 3

What is Holistic Care?

According to *Taber's Cyclopedic Medical Dictionary*, holistic medicine refers to the "comprehensive and total care of a patient. In this system, the needs of the patient in all areas, such as physical, emotional, social, spiritual, and economic, are considered and cared for."

If asked, most hospice professionals will tell you that caring for terminally ill patients and their families is not so much a choice, but a "calling." I have met nurses working in this specialty that felt differently and soon left for another type of nursing. The ones who have persevered for many years tell me that although it is physically demanding, mentally and emotionally exhausting, and, at times, spiritually challenging, they stay—not so much out of want, but out of need.

They know their patients have no hope of being cured. They know many of their patients are afraid to die but are more afraid to live in pain. They know they will not be able to heal those in their care, but they need to comfort them anyway. These nurses need to laugh with their patients, cry with them, talk to them, and listen to them. And when their dying patients are feeling abandoned and alone, they need to sit in a quiet room and hold their hands. It is nurses like these who administer holistic care that keep the ever-expanding hospice movement closely connected to its roots. In fact, many families become so fond of the hospice nurse that after the death of their family member they experience a "secondary loss" due to no longer receiving visits from the nurse who lovingly cared for them as well.

Hospice care encompasses holistic care. It is a personal approach to the total care of one who is facing impending death. Hospice professionals view the patient, family, and caregivers as one unit to be looked after and comforted. They care for the physical pain of the patient, the emotional and mental anguish of the patient and family, and the spiritual conflicts that often arise within the patient and family members. As caregivers, we also have the opportunity to perform the same service.

Relieving the patient's physical pain is foremost. Only when pain is relieved and symptoms are controlled can other levels of consciousness be soothed. One who is experiencing excruciating bone pain from cancer, for example, cannot concentrate on why she is afraid of dying. Once she feels some relief from the physical pain, her other work can begin. As a caregiver, in-depth communication with your patient cannot begin until he is physically comfortable. It also cannot begin until you have started to examine your own thoughts and feelings about the situation that is confronting you. You may not reach concrete conclusions at this early stage, but it is here that the journey begins. Whether you are caring for a family member, friend, senior Vaishnava, godbrother or godsister, you cannot help but experience a sense of loss as each day passes. Once death occurs for the devotee, you will no longer have his personal association. That sense of emptiness and grief begins to unfold a long time before the devotee passes away. By Krishna's grace, we are allowed this time to prepare for the unavoidable. Because the Lord promises to carry what we lack and preserve what we have, He strengthens us for when we will need it the most.

What is Spiritual Pain?

Because grieving starts a long time before the actual death experience, the patient, family, and caregivers may experience what is called "anticipatory grief." This occurs when family members and close friends realize that death of their loved one is unavoidable. This occurs for the patient when he realizes that his life will end much sooner than expected. Anticipatory grief is sometimes referred to as "pre-death" bereavement. As a caregiver you need to give your patient, as well as yourself, permission to grieve.

Spiritual pain can be intensely private and can manifest itself in many ways. Perhaps the dying devotee did not accomplish what he wanted to in life. Perhaps his children are not yet grown and he worries what will become of them or if they will even remember him. Perhaps there was a particular service he wanted to perform for his spiritual master and now that is impossible. A devotee may regret having wasted so much time when not engaged in devotional service. When someone is very ill, with months—or even weeks—to live, remembering one moment that was wasted can cause mental anguish, guilt, and regret.

Unexpected emotions can often manifest in one who is facing imminent death. The patient may even vacillate between feeling spiritually strong one day and emotionally weak and vulnerable the next. This is common. When someone is experiencing spiritual pain she may cry, become anxious, or exhibit anger at seemingly inappropriate times. She may even joke about dying, which is often a way to mask her fear and anxiety.

We can help by becoming good listeners. Being in the presence of a sensitive listener will enable the devotee to release some of her anxieties, even if that anxiety stems from fearing the pain associated with the dying process. We must not hear with judgmental minds, but with compassionate hearts. We can help by creating an atmosphere of safe boundaries so the devotee, if willing, can comfortably reveal her mind and reach emotionally sound and Krishna-conscious conclusions.

Therefore, as much as the dying devotee will allow, this time can be seen as a window of opportunity to increase your intimate relationship in a mood of Krishna consciousness. The dying devotee must not fear being ridiculed. Choosing each word carefully, saying what you feel, asking what you can do for him, and expressing your gratitude for having known him will create a mood of love and trust in which he can reciprocate. This is the time to share spiritual realizations and to reassure the dying devotee that the Lord will never leave him. I once heard a senior devotee in our movement say, "Krishna is not an ingrate. He will never forget the service you have rendered. He will never abandon you."

Certainly this is true of the dying devotee who has taken shelter of the Lord. As a caregiver, you have a tremendous opportunity to remind the devotee of this truth.

How Can the Caregiver Help?

Even if bedridden, when a devotee is encouraged to engage in devotional service to the Lord, any spiritual anxieties he may have will soon be diminished. Gently remind him of what Prahlad Maharaja said in the *Srimad-Bhagavatam*: "Hearing and chanting about the transcendental holy name, form, qualities, paraphernalia, and pastimes of Lord Vishnu, remembering them, serving the lotus feet of the Lord, offering the Lord respectful worship with sixteen types of paraphernalia, offering prayers to the Lord, becoming His servant, considering the Lord one's best friend, and surrendering everything unto Him—these nine processes are accepted as pure devotional service. One who has dedicated his life to the service of Krishna through these nine methods should be understood to be the most learned person, for he has acquired complete knowledge." (SB 7.5.24)

In this regard, in his Introduction to the *Bhagavad-gita As It Is*, Srila Prabhupada writes:

> If one has fifty years of life ahead of him, he should engage that brief time in cultivating this practice of remembering the Supreme Personality of Godhead. This practice is the devotional process of:
>
> *sravanam kirtanam visnoh smaranam pada sevanam*
> *arcanam vandanam dasyam sakhyam atma-nivedanam*
>
> These nine processes, of which the easiest is *sravanam*, hearing *Bhagavad-gita* from the realized person, will turn one to the thought of the Supreme Being. This will lead to *niscala*, remembering the Supreme Lord, and will enable one, upon leaving the body, to attain a spiritual body which is just fit for association with the Supreme Lord.

Here, Srila Prabhupada refers to another fifty years of life as a "brief time." If one is aware that death will come in only a few months, he may feel a sense of spiritual urgency that may cause anxiety and could lead to spiritual pain. Remind him that the nine processes of devotional service can be performed in spite of the body's diseased condition. As a caregiver, support him in whatever service he desires to render. If he is physically incapable of performing a service, you can offer to do it under his guidance so he will not only be a participant but a teacher as well. This will give the devotee a feeling that he is passing on his knowledge of devotional service to others. This sense of "handing down" knowledge as a kind of legacy is essential for a terminally ill patient as he assesses his life. The hospice philosophy of dying with dignity allows for every person to feel that his life has brought value to the world and that his wisdom will not be forgotten. By the grace of the *guru*, devotees possess the greatest knowledge. Allow for the dying Vaishnava to transmit that wisdom to those he will leave behind.

As someone's condition begins to worsen, she may only be able to read, chant, or even speak for short periods of time. Your patient will require more rest as the disease takes control of her body. Staying awake will become difficult. Pacing these devotional activities will help to avoid fatigue. The following suggestions may help you with your tremendous task of assisting the devotee spiritually during her final journey:

- For some, chanting the Hare Krishna *mantra* on *japa* beads may be feasible when first diagnosed but may become increasingly difficult or even impossible, depending on the disease process. If he is able to verbalize but is no longer able to manipulate *japa* beads, ask if you can place his beads in his right hand so he can feel them, sit at his bedside, and chant the Hare Krishna *mantra* so he can chant with you. If he eventually becomes unresponsive, this can still be performed. Hearing is the last sense to leave us. Rest assured that the devotee will still hear you chanting.

- Ask your patient if she would like to hear a recording of Srila Prabhupada chanting *japa*. Or perhaps she would like to meditate on the Lord while hearing Srila Prabhupada chant a soft *bhajan*.

- Provide the devotee with the opportunity to hear a lecture recording. If available, ask him if he would like to listen to class using earphones to increase concentration. Eventually he may become too weak to remove the earphones by himself. Remove them occasionally for comfort or if he needs to rest.

- Offer to have devotees visit to have a *kirtan* or sing *bhajans*. Someone who is terminally ill, however, may become increasingly sensitive to loud sound. Ask her if she prefers a peaceful *bhajan* as opposed to a louder *kirtan*. Be aware of the volume of any musical instruments, such as a *mrdanga* drum or *karatals* (cymbals).

- Discuss Lord Krishna's transcendental pastimes in Vrindavan.

- Glorify the pastimes of Lord Chaitanya Mahaprabhu.

- Exchange realizations about Srila Prabhupada's unlimited compassion for the conditioned souls and his determination to fulfill the orders of his Guru Maharaja. This will also provide an opportunity for the dying Vaishnava to reflect on his own life and what might have happened if he had never met Srila Prabhupada or the devotees of His Divine Grace. This type of self-reflection not only increases one's appreciation for Srila Prabhupada and the society of Vaishnavas, but also assists the devotee in reviewing his own life, a necessary tool in reaching an emotional and mental closure before dying.

- Ask the devotee if you can read aloud the translations to some of the songs written by Srila Narottama Dasa Thakura, Srila Bhaktivinoda Thakura, and other Vaishnava *acharyas* who provided us with poetic prayers upon which to meditate.

- Ask your patient if she would like to view a Krishna-conscious video.

- Ask him if he would like to read Srila Prabhupada's books silently, or if you can read them aloud to him.

- If the devotee is being cared for in a temple, or if she can easily be transported to a nearby temple, ask her if she wishes to take *darshan* of the Deities.

- If he has household Deities ask if you can assist him in Their worship. Help him to serve Their Lordships in any way he wishes. Be aware that smoke caused by cooking or burning incense may cause respiratory difficulties or even nausea. (Caution: If an oxygen tank or concentrator is in use, be sure to avoid open flames such as candles, ghee lamps, the lighting of incense, etc. Please note that the burning of incense may exacerbate breathing difficulties for some patients.)

As the devotee's terminal condition progresses, he may eventually become nonverbal and unresponsive. His devotional service will not end here. Although he will not be able to respond, he will still be able to hear transcendental sound vibration, chant the *maha-mantra* within his mind, remember the pastimes of Krishna, offer prayers to Krishna, and meditate on serving the Lord. Toward the end of his life it may appear externally that your patient is in a coma-like state, but internally he will be doing a great deal of work. You can facilitate his devotional service by reading scripture to him, softly chanting by his side, or keeping quiet chanting or a lecture playing within hearing range. If he has not expressed it sooner, it should be assumed that at this stage of his disease process he may be sensitive not only to loud volume but to bright light. Provide a calm environment with soft transcendental sounds, natural lighting during the day, and diffuse light in the evening.

However, while your patient is still able to verbalize her wishes, allow her the freedom to choose when she wants to hear scripture, when she wants to hear chanting, or when she wishes for silence. It is best to ask her whether she wants to see visitors, be with caregivers, or simply be alone. Respect her desires and you will be doing a great service for this courageous Vaishnava.

Communicating with One Who is Dying

Be sure the patient wants to talk with someone

It is not always easy or comfortable speaking to someone who is terminally ill. Even the most well-meaning intentions can go awry when we approach a patient thinking he wants to engage in a deep conversation about his situation only to find he does not. Often the patient is physically tired or has just had an intense conversation that has left him emotionally exhausted. He simply may not be in the mood to discuss something so multifaceted. At times, he may feel frustrated thinking no one can possibly understand what he is going through. This frustration may lead to angry outbursts. Even the most well-meaning friend or family member can seem like an intruder to the patient when he does not wish to engage in an intense conversation. Although a terminal illness affects everyone associated with the patient, ultimately it is the patient alone who is facing what seems to be an "untimely death." Even a devotee needs to go through a kind of "mental processing period" to come to terms with her life being suddenly cut short. Discussing her situation with someone may or may not assist her in this process. How she spends her last remaining days searching for conclusions will be her choice and her right. As a caregiver, you need to remind yourself and others that the patient will, most likely, want to talk at another time. For now, ask her if she wants to be alone. If so, allow her that simple comfort. If she states that she does not want to be alone, but does not want to engage in conversation either, ask her if you can sit by her side without speaking. If you feel at ease with the silence, so will she.

Concentrate on the patient, not on yourself

Often, when having a conversation, we seem to be listening to what the other person is saying but do not really hear him. This may occur because we are preoccupied with our own responses or because we are looking for what we want to hear. The latter frequently occurs when speaking with a terminally-ill patient, especially one we care about very much. As a caregiver to a devotee, you will naturally want your patient or loved one to reach the Krishna-conscious conclusions you feel he needs in order to attain spiritual peace. We may be so anxious for the dying devotee to have the realizations we desire for him that we do not truly hear what he is actually expressing. Spiritual awareness must be nurtured, never rushed. Allow your listening to facilitate another's communication. Let your attitude reflect the privilege of listening. Hear what he is trying to communicate to you and not what you want him to say.

Avoid giving advice unless you are asked

When speaking to a terminally-ill patient, it is not recommended to begin a sentence with, "If I were you I would…" This may very well put a halt to your conversation. The patient may respond by saying, "But you are not me," and he would be justified in responding this way. After all, we cannot fully comprehend what a dying person is experiencing. We can empathize, but until we are in a similar situation it is difficult to fully understand. Still, we can try to put ourselves in the place of the patient, always reminding ourselves to separate our needs from his. If you are asked for advice and do not know what to say, be honest. Tell him that you do not truly understand what he is experiencing. If you would like to offer advice, you may want to begin your suggestions with sensitive phrases like "Have you ever considered..." or "What do you think about..." Perhaps the dying devotee does not want advice. He knows what he must do. He may simply want the comfort of knowing that someone understands his unique pain.

Reassure the devotee that his life has made a difference in the world

As previously discussed, every person deserves to feel that his life has had meaning and worth. He needs to know that he has contributed something valuable to the world, to his family members, to his friends, and to his godbrothers and godsisters. As a devotee, your patient has made more of a difference than he probably realizes. Remind him that he will not be forgotten by family, friends, or by the society of devotees. Speaking from your heart, tell him that you are a better person and a better devotee having known him. If you do not tell him now, you may never have the opportunity again.

Be prepared to cover the same subject matter again and again

Sometimes a terminally-ill patient may need to verbalize the same thoughts, realizations, anxieties, or fears many times before she can move on. Do not feel guilty if you feel a bit frustrated at hearing the same points repeated over and over again by your patient. She may even need to hear you repeat the same answers you have told her many times before. Although this repetition can be wearisome to the caregiver, it is sometimes necessary for the patient. Those who are coping with tremendous emotional stress may need to repeatedly cover the same subjects until they are comfortable with their conclusions. Helping someone who is dying can be both humbling and exhausting, but it is the most valuable thing you can ever do for someone.

Remember to paraphrase the patient's statements

This technique involves stating in your own words what you think someone just said. Paraphrasing reassures the patient that you are not only listening to what he is saying, but are truly attempting to understand him. You may want to start a sentence by saying, "What I hear you saying is..." or "In other words..." or "So what you are telling me is..." Use this technique whenever the devotee says something that seems important to him, and he will appreciate your effort to understand him.

Don't be afraid to ask important questions

If you feel your patient wants to talk about her situation but feels awkward getting the conversation started, you may want to ask some of the following questions:

- What is this experience like for you?
- How is your family reacting to this?
- Are you feeling afraid?
- How can I help?
- How do you want to spend this time?
- Do you have any regrets or unfinished business?
- Can I help you arrange anything?
- Do you want anyone in particular to visit you?
- What have you learned from all of this?
- What spiritual realizations have you had since being diagnosed?

If the devotee reacts as if you have invaded his privacy by asking some of these questions, you can always apologize and back away from these sensitive issues. He may not be ready to discuss these things, or discussing them at another time might be more appropriate.

Remember the importance of nonverbal communication

Although a person may articulate something, his or her body language may convey a different message. Body language can be described as "clusters of signals that convey information." Often, when spoken words and body language are different, the nonverbal message is what is communicated. ("He told me he had read the book, but I didn't believe him.") Also, nonverbal signals are interpreted differently according to cultural variations. Below are some nonverbal cues that may decrease communication:

- Poor eye contact (looking away or closing eyes for more than a second)

- Body turned away (depicts disinterest)

- Feet turned away (if standing, depicts disinterest)

- Sitting behind a desk or other barrier (depicts wanting to distance ourselves)

- Holding a barrier in front of the body (if standing, depicts wanting to distance ourselves)

- Arms folded across chest (depicts defensiveness or wanting to distance ourselves)

- Clenched fists (depicts anger or defensiveness)

- Shifting weight from one foot to the other (depicts awkwardness)

- Rubbing neck (depicts criticism)

- Fidgeting with clothes or other objects (depicts nervousness)

- Peering over eyeglasses (depicts a judgmental attitude)

- Wringing of hands (depicts nervousness or frustration)

On the contrary, we can send powerful, positive messages with our body language. For example, sitting down with someone on his or her physical level shows you care and are interested in what is being said. Leaning slightly forward indicates that you are giving him your complete attention. Similarly, we tend to turn toward something or someone who interests us. Nodding while she is speaking will show you understand what she is trying to convey. It does not always mean that you necessarily agree with the speaker.

Touch, when used appropriately, can send a message of caring and support. It also improves trust between the patient and caregiver. A light touch on your patient's hand, for instance, can communicate empathy when he may need it the most. Several studies have shown that touch can have strong therapeutic value and can offer psychological and physical comfort. I have had patients, however, that experienced such excruciating pain that even a light touch on the hand hurt them. Be aware of what your patient can tolerate. Touch is also interpreted in various ways according to different cultures. A warm smile is universal and always suggests kindness and compassion.

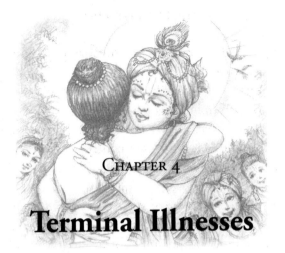

Chapter 4

Terminal Illnesses

In this chapter, many diseases are discussed which, at their end stage, are considered terminal and hospice-appropriate. This discussion only briefly refers to some terminal illnesses and is not meant to be all-inclusive. It is, however, meant to prompt further inquiry by the reader, if desired.

Acquired Immune Deficiency Syndrome (AIDS)

Acquired Immune Deficiency Syndrome (AIDS) is a syndrome of opportunistic infections that occur as the result of uncontrolled spread of the human immunodeficiency virus (HIV). When the virus is uncontrolled, these opportunistic diseases can invade every system of the body and eventually cause death. The Center for Disease Control and Prevention (CDC) first described the virus in 1981. HIV is spread by intimate sexual contact, contaminated needles or blood products, or from mother to child. Blood products are now routinely screened to prevent transmission of the virus through blood transfusions.

When contracted, HIV attaches itself to cells in the body, specifically the CD4 receptors of T-cells. T-cells are lymphocytes (white blood cells) that fight infection. HIV can infect other cells with CD4 receptors, as well. Once attached, the virus then enters the cells, infiltrates the ribonucleic acid (RNA), transfers its own deoxyribonucleic acid (DNA) to the cells, and prevents the cells from performing their normal function. With the transfer of its own DNA, the virus can then replicate. Diagnosis of HIV is determined by a simple blood test that detects antibodies that the body naturally develops to fight the virus. Antibodies to HIV can usually be detected approximately two to six weeks after exposure to the virus. Early symptoms may include a mild fever, muscular pain, joint pain, weight loss, and rash. Even when an HIV-infected person has no symptoms, he can still infect others and should be under the care of a physician.

Highly active antiretroviral agents (HAART), medications introduced in 1996 to fight HIV, have greatly reduced the number of opportunistic infections contracted by HIV-infected patients. Each type of drug works on a different part of the replication cycle of the virus. When taken in combination, they have proven to suppress viral replication for long periods of time. In a 1996 issue of the *New England Journal of Medicine*, it states, "The goal of antiretroviral therapy should be to reduce levels of circulating virus as much as possible, for as long as possible." For those who have access to these medications and are able to follow a strict daily regime, the HIV infection has now become more of a chronic long-term disease.

It's important to note, however, that these medications are not a cure for HIV or AIDS, and those undergoing this medication regime may still develop infections. They also have not been shown to eliminate the risk of passing HIV to others through sexual contact or blood contamination. Those who are undiagnosed, untreated, not properly treated, or those for whom antiretroviral therapy has failed are still at risk of developing many of the opportunistic infections long associated with AIDS. The development of these opportunistic infections, as well as the number of T4 cells in the body, signals the difference between being HIV-infected and having AIDS. Those patients who do not comply with their medication regime, those who do not have access to HAART, and those in third-world countries are at additional risk for developing AIDS.

There are many opportunistic illnesses that can compromise the health of a person infected with HIV. The ones listed below are among the most common.

- **Pneumocystis carinii pneumonia (PCP)** — A lung infection caused by an organism found in air, food, and water. It is the most common lung infection found in patients with AIDS. Symptoms include fever, fatigue, shortness of breath, and persistent cough. An HIV-infected patient with a T4 cell count below 200 has an increased chance of developing PCP.

- **Toxoplasmosis** — A disease of the brain caused by an organism found in, among other sources, vegetables and unpasteurized dairy products. The illness can be transmitted from mother to fetus through the umbilical cord if acquired during pregnancy. This disease affects the central nervous system (CNS), causing headaches, seizures, confusion, memory loss, one-sided paralysis, visual defects, absence or impairment of speech, and impaired muscle coordination.

- **Mycobacterium Avium-Intracellular (MAI) Infection** — This infection is caused by bacteria found in soil, air, water, raw dairy products, and other environmental sources. It rarely causes infection in healthy individuals, but in a person with AIDS it may affect the blood, lymph nodes, bone marrow, liver, lungs, and gastrointestinal tract. Symptoms often include fever, severe diarrhea, weight loss, fatigue, fever, abdominal pain, and night sweats.

- **Herpes Simplex Virus** — This is a chronic infection caused by a herpes virus and is commonly seen in patients with AIDS. Herpes Simplex 1 is spread through oral secretions. Symptoms include painful blister-like lesions on the lips, tongue, or inside the mouth. In patients with AIDS, lesions may spread to the esophagus, trachea, and lungs. Herpes Simplex 2 is spread through intimate sexual contact causing lesions in the genital area. Other symptoms can include fever and fatigue. In patients with AIDS, this infection can cause complications such as bronchitis, esophagitis (inflammation of the esophagus), pericarditis (inflammation of the sac that encloses the heart), and encephalitis (inflammation of the brain).

- **Cytomegalovirus (CMV) Infection** — CMV is one of the herpes viruses. In patients with compromised immune systems, it can affect the lungs, central nervous system, eyes, gastrointestinal tract, adrenal glands, and blood. Symptoms can include fever, swollen lymph nodes, enlarged liver and spleen, stomach and intestinal ulcers, and blindness.

- **Candida Albicans Infection** — This is a disease caused by a fungus. It is most commonly found in the mouth, throat, and esophagus. It is characterized by the presence of white patches in the mouth and difficulty swallowing. This infection is common among patients with AIDS.

- **Progressive Multifocal Leukoencephalopathy (PML)** — PML is an illness affecting the central nervous system. It is caused by the papovavirus and causes gradual brain degeneration. Symptoms can include confusion, headache, seizures, visual loss, weakened limbs, speech disturbances, and lethargy. In advanced stages it can cause partial paralysis and coma.

Alzheimer's Disease

In general, many people do not think of Alzheimer's disease as a terminal illness, but in its final stages it is considered a hospice-appropriate disease. It is the most common cause of dementia (a progressive condition causing, among other things, intellectual impairment, memory loss, apathy, and speech disturbances), contributing to about 50% of all cases. Because it is progressive, prognosis is poor. Duration of the disease generally lasts from three to 20 years, with an average of approximately seven years from diagnosis to death. It is rarely seen in patients before 45 years of age.

Alzheimer's disease causes irreversible damage to brain cells, causing early symptoms of short-term memory loss, forgetfulness, inability to concentrate, difficulty learning new information, and often, deterioration in personal hygiene. In its later stages, Alzheimer's disease may cause deterioration of long-term memory and communication, including spoken and written language; repetitive actions; urinary and fecal incontinence; and personality changes, including extreme agitation that can lead to violent episodes. In its final stage, patients with Alzheimer's disease often stop eating and drinking, leading to dehydration and starvation. They are also at high risk for infections, a major cause of death. Because of decreased mobility, many patients are at risk for decubitus ulcers (sometimes referred to as bed sores or pressure sores). Usually occurring over bony areas of the body, decubitus ulcers can begin with superficial skin maceration or become deep enough to expose muscle and even bone. Meticulous skin care as well as frequent repositioning of a patient with Alzheimer's disease (at least every two hours round the clock) is essential to help avoid such ulcers.

Being a caregiver of a patient with Alzheimer's disease can be physically and emotionally wearing. Caregivers require a great deal of support from family and friends, with regular relief for rest.

The cause of Alzheimer's disease is still unknown, although research is ongoing. New medications are now available that can slow its progression in some patients who are in the early stages of the disease. However, the illness still remains irreversible.

Diagnosis is difficult. Tests involve physical and neuropsychological testing which tests memory, reasoning, language ability, and vision-motor coordination. Often a psychiatric evaluation is done. A magnetic resonance imaging (MRI) study of the brain is used to search for other possible reasons for dementia, such as a tumor or a stroke. Blood tests are also performed. As of this writing, a definite diagnosis of Alzheimer's disease cannot be made until autopsy, because microscopic examination of brain tissue is required. Some families choose to have this performed after the patient's death as a means to provide family medical history.

Amyotrophic Lateral Sclerosis

Amyotrophic Lateral Sclerosis (ALS) was first written about in the late 1800s, but became known as Lou Gehrig's disease in 1939 when the famous New York Yankee showed great courage after being diagnosed with the illness. ALS is a neurological disease caused by the degeneration of upper and lower motor neurons in a part of the brain called the medulla oblongata and the spinal cord. It leads to progressive muscular weakness and the inability to speak and, eventually, to swallow. The disease progresses rapidly in some patients and slowly in others. It often begins in the limbs with muscle weakness but can start with speech and swallowing difficulties. The incidence of onset is usually between the ages of 50 and 70. It is rare under the age of 30. ALS leads to quadriplegia (paralysis of all limbs) and to a loss of speech, swallowing, and eventually, the ability to breathe.

Patients with ALS usually remain mentally alert through their illness, since it does not affect intellect. Similarly, ALS does not affect eyesight, hearing, or bladder and bowel control. It can sometimes affect emotions, causing a patient to laugh or cry at inappropriate times. The life of an ALS patient becomes extremely limiting and often frustrating, since complete care, such as bathing, dressing, feeding, turning, and lifting is eventually required. (It is essential that the primary caregiver be relieved at regular intervals in order to receive adequate emotional and physical rest.)

When the patient can no longer speak or move his limbs, communication becomes difficult. Boredom and loneliness are common. Communication devices such as a word board or picture board can be helpful. A caregiver points to a word or picture while the patient blinks his eyes to confirm. This system can be tedious, but effective. I once cared for a young man with ALS who wrote an entire book of poems using a laptop computer and a special device that was clipped to his eyeglasses. He blinked on each letter that then typed itself onto the screen. In this way, this gentleman of 46 years of age, determined to leave something behind after his death, patiently typed each word of each sentence and eventually wrote an entire volume of poetry.

The average prognosis is two to five years after diagnosis, although I cared for hospice patients who died after having ALS for eight to ten years. In patients who choose palliative care at the end stage of this disease, death usually occurs from respiratory failure. When patients choose aggressive treatment, such as the use of a ventilator, death usually comes from pneumonia.

Initial symptoms may include slurred speech, uncontrolled drooling, hand weakness, muscle twitching, poor balance when standing or walking causing frequent falls, and shortness of breath on exertion. Diagnosis is made after a physical examination, study of clinical symptoms, and exclusion of other possible causes for the symptoms. More invasive testing to confirm a diagnosis of ALS may include electromyography, blood tests, nerve conduction studies, muscle biopsy, and examination of cerebrospinal fluid.

Cancer

There are an estimated 200 different types of cancer. All forms of cancer involve the uncontrolled growth of abnormal cells derived from normal tissue. Even when discovered in its early stages, these cells may or may not spread. When they do spread, it is called metastasis. Unfortunately, many cancers remain silent, with few or no symptoms at first, so by the time they are discovered they may have already metastasized to other parts of the body. Benign tumors are not cancer. They can usually be removed and, in most cases, do not return. The cells in benign tumors do not spread and, therefore, are not life-threatening. On the other hand, malignant tumor cells are cancerous and can break away from the original tumor.

Normally, cells in the body grow, divide, and eventually die in a systematic order. As we reach adulthood, this process slows and most cells divide only to restore worn-out cells or to repair injuries. Cancer cells continue to grow and divide, however, and when gathered together, form tumors that invade normal tissue. When cells break away from the original tumor, they can travel through the bloodstream or the lymphatic system. They are then free to compress and invade other parts of the body, including major organs. Even when a particular type of cancer has spread, it is still referred to by its original or primary site of growth. For example, if a patient has breast cancer that metastasizes to the lungs, it is still called breast cancer, or metastatic breast cancer.

Various types of cancer cells differ in their growth, pattern of spread, and response to treatment. Pain caused by various types of cancer responds to different pain medications, as well. For instance, what alleviates pain for some patients with bone cancer may not be effective for someone with bladder cancer.

"Staging" refers to the extent and prognosis of the tumor. There are many staging systems of cancer. A common system is the tumor, node, and metastasis system (TNM) that adds numbers to each of these categories, depending on the distribution of the cancer cells.

Some important warning signs of cancer to be aware of are:

- Unusual bleeding or discharge, either internally or externally

- Any lump or thickening

- A sore that does not heal

- A significant change of bowel or bladder habits

- A persistent cough or hoarseness

- Difficulty swallowing

- The appearance of a new wart or mole, or a change in size and shape of an existing wart or mole

- Unexplained weight loss

Any of these signs should immediately be brought to the attention of a physician. Diagnosis is made by various means, such as biopsy, computerized tomography (CT scan), mammography, or ultrasound, depending on the site of the suspected cancer.

Cerebrovascular Disease (CVA)

Cerebrovascular disease (CVA) is also referred to as a stroke. A stroke most commonly occurs when a blood clot blocks an artery carrying blood to the brain, or when one of these blood vessels breaks. In either case, blood flow to a portion of the brain is interrupted; therefore oxygen to that part of the brain ceases as well. Within minutes or a few hours after a stroke begins, the brain cells in the immediate area die. This area of dead brain cells is called an infarct. The dead cells then release a chemical that creates a type of chain reaction that kills cells in surrounding areas of the brain, where blood flow is compromised but not completely blocked. This chain reaction occurs quickly. Therefore, it is believed that the first six hours after stroke symptoms occur is crucial for medical intervention. Once the stroke begins, every second counts in order to increase one's chances of recovery. Some risk factors include: diabetes mellitus, hypertension (high blood pressure), arteriosclerosis (a thickening and hardening of the artery walls), gout, increased triglyceride levels, family history of CVA, decreased exercise, use of oral contraceptives, and cigarette smoking.

A patient will develop loss of certain abilities depending on which part of the brain is affected by the stroke, as well as the size of the area of dead cells. Loss of function may involve movement, speech, and memory. A small stroke may leave only weakness in an arm and leg, for example, whereas a larger stroke may leave one paralyzed and unable to speak. If a stroke occurs on the left side of the brain, the right side of the body is affected. If it occurs on the right side of the brain, symptoms occur on the left side of the body. CVA is the third most common cause of death in the United States, attacking mostly older adults. It can, however, occur at any age. Diagnostic tests include computed tomography (CT) scan of the brain, a lumbar puncture (spinal puncture), an electroencephalogram (EEG), and an angiogram.

Chronic Obstructive Pulmonary Disease

Chronic Obstructive Pulmonary Disease (COPD) is an airway obstruction that can result from many conditions such as emphysema, chronic bronchitis, cystic fibrosis, or asthma. Often a patient may suffer from more than one of these illnesses before COPD develops. It is a chronic condition that tends to worsen with time. Cigarette smokers are at high risk for developing COPD. Chronic lung infections and allergies may also contribute to the disease.

Symptoms can include a chronic cough, shortness of breath on minimal exertion, an anxious feeling, audible wheezing, tachypnea (rapid respirations), and tachycardia (rapid heartbeat). Diagnostic tests for COPD include a chest x-ray, pulmonary function tests, blood tests, and an EKG. In end-stage COPD, patients generally require constant oxygen therapy and may have extreme difficulty breathing even when in a sitting position. Understandably, patients with advanced chronic obstructive pulmonary disease usually exhibit a tremendous amount of anxiety.

Congestive Heart Failure

Congestive heart failure (CHF) is a disease in which the heart becomes inefficient and cannot pump enough blood to meet the demands of the body's organs. As blood flows too slowly from the heart due to diminished cardiac output, the blood returning to the heart backs up and causes congestion in the tissues. As a result, edema (swelling) can occur, usually in the patient's legs and feet. Fluid can also form in the lungs, which can cause breathing difficulty. (Pulmonary edema is an acute, life-threatening condition.) Congestive heart failure can cause the kidneys to inadequately rid the body of sodium and water, a condition that also contributes to edema. CHF often occurs on the left side of the heart but can also develop in the right side. Sometimes, left- and right-sided heart failure can occur simultaneously.

Symptoms of CHF differ according to which side of the heart is affected. For example, left-sided heart failure may cause dyspnea (difficulty breathing), tachycardia (rapid heartbeat), edema, weight gain, fatigue, and muscle weakness. Right-sided heart failure may cause edema, distended neck veins, and hepatomegaly (an enlarged liver).

There are many causes of congestive heart failure. Some common causes include coronary artery disease (the narrowing of arteries that supply blood to the heart), myocardial infarction (a previous heart attack that leaves scar tissue to interfere with the heart muscle), hypertension (high blood pressure), previous rheumatic fever, congenital heart disease (heart defects present at birth), and infections of the heart valves or muscle, such as endocarditis or myocarditis. Diagnostic tests to determine if someone has congestive heart failure may include a chest x-ray, an EKG, cardiac catheterization, and an echocardiogram. Prognosis of the disease depends on the cause and its response to treatment.

Diabetes Mellitus

Diabetes mellitus is a chronic disease caused by inadequate production of insulin or the inability to utilize the insulin produced. Both men and women are equally affected. The incidence rises with age.

Type I diabetes refers to a condition in which a person secretes little or no insulin. This is also called insulin-dependent diabetes mellitus (IDDM). In the past, it was referred to as juvenile diabetes. IDDM usually occurs before age 30, although it can occur at any age. In Type II diabetes, or non-insulin dependent diabetes (NIDDM), a patient develops insulin resistance or insufficiency. It is sometimes called adult-onset diabetes and usually occurs in patients after age 40. It is most frequently treated with diet and exercise, although oral hypoglycemia medications may be required. Type II diabetes is more common than Type I. Diabetes causes disturbances in the metabolism of carbohydrates, protein, and fat. It is a chronic, incurable disease, but symptoms can be controlled with proper therapy.

Hereditary factors play a key role in developing diabetes. Other causes that may attribute to the disease include obesity; physiologic or emotional stress that causes prolonged elevation of stress hormones resulting in elevated blood glucose levels which increase demands on the pancreas (the organ that helps produce insulin); pregnancy that increases levels of estrogen and placental hormones; and certain medications that are known to antagonize the effects of insulin.

Patients with diabetes mellitus are at risk for two very serious metabolic complications caused by hyperglycemia (increased blood sugar levels) called diabetic ketoacidosis (DKA) and hyperosmolar nonketotic syndrome (HNKS). These are acute, life-threatening conditions that can lead to dehydration, shock, coma, and death, and they therefore require immediate medical attention. Diabetic patients are also at risk for developing chronic illnesses such as cardiovascular disease, peripheral vascular disease (often leading to amputation of lower limbs), severe hypertension (increased blood pressure), retinopathy (a disorder of the retina that can lead to blindness), nephropathy (a disease of the kidneys), and peripheral neuropathy (a disease of the nerves usually causing pain and numbness in the hands and feet).

Signs and symptoms of diabetes mellitus may include weakness or fatigue, polyuria (increased urination), polydypsia (excessive thirst), dry mucous membranes, weight loss in IDDM, and polyphagia (eating excessive amounts of food) in IDDM. Diagnostic tests include various blood and urine tests.

Occasionally, hospice patients with cancer of the pancreas may develop diabetes secondary to their cancer. In any hospice patient with diabetes, care is taken to avoid hyperglycemia (increased levels of blood sugar) or hypoglycemia (decreased levels of blood sugar). Symptoms of hypoglycemia include headaches, confusion, dizziness, sweating, irritability, or tremors. If not treated, hypoglycemia can lead to seizures and coma. Signs and symptoms of hyperglycemia may include excessive thirst, frequent urination, fatigue, weakness, abdominal pain, nausea, vomiting, fruity breath, drowsiness, flushed skin, and general discomfort. If a diabetic patient was taking insulin medications prior to his hospice admission, it is generally continued even if the patient stops eating because the liver continues to produce glucose. Once the patient becomes unresponsive (unconscious), insulin is usually stopped in hospice care.

Hepatitis

Hepatitis is a disease causing inflammation of the liver. There are many types of hepatitis viruses, some with higher risk of complications than others. Hepatitis may be acute, meaning it has a sudden onset with severe symptoms, but runs a short course. Hepatitis may also be chronic, meaning it is of long duration and/or slow progression. Patients with chronic hepatitis are at risk of lasting liver disease. This can be of a serious nature, because the liver has many functions, including:

- Storing iron, vitamins, and minerals
- Producing bile to help in digestion
- Acting as a filter to convert poisonous chemicals to substances that can either be used by the body or excreted from the body
- Converting food into stored energy
- Producing new proteins
- Producing clotting factors so blood can clot

Types of Viral Hepatitis

Hepatitis A, formerly known as infectious hepatitis, is highly contagious. It is transmitted by the fecal to oral route. It can result from ingesting contaminated milk, food, or water. The hepatitis A virus enters the digestive tract and begins reproducing. It then spreads to the liver and multiplies in the liver cells. The incubation period (the amount of time between infection and the development of symptoms) is usually two to four weeks. Symptoms may include fatigue, abdominal pain, decreased appetite, nausea, diarrhea, and jaundice in which the skin and the whites of the eyes become yellowish. A complication that can occur with hepatitis A is a relapse after apparent recovery. If desired, a vaccine is available for long-term prevention of hepatitis A virus infection for those two years of age and older.

Hepatitis B virus is transmitted through exchange of contaminated blood, intimate sexual contact, contact with contaminated bodily secretions and feces, and from mother to child. The hepatitis B virus can cause lifelong infections, cirrhosis (scarring) of the liver, liver cancer, liver failure, and death. The average incubation period for hepatitis B is two to three months. Initial symptoms may resemble the flu: fatigue, abdominal discomfort, fever, decreased appetite, nausea, and diarrhea. Other symptoms include dark urine, pale stools, and jaundice (yellowish eyes and skin). Invasive diagnostic testing includes a blood test and sometimes a needle biopsy of the liver to test for the virus and liver damage. In general, hepatitis B is treated over a period of four months with a medication called interferon that is given by injection. In advanced stages where liver function ceases, a liver transplant may be needed. A three-step vaccine is available for all age groups to prevent the virus. Healthcare workers are at increased risk of being infected by hepatitis B due to the presence of infectious materials in their work place. In some countries, including the United States, the three-step vaccine is mandatory for all employees working in healthcare facilities.

Hepatitis C (HCV) is transmitted through contaminated blood and bodily fluids, from mother to child, as well as intravenous drug use (presently the most common type of transmission). It is now known that hepatitis C is rarely transmitted sexually and studies show that sexual transmissions account for less than 5% of cases. Even with such a small percentage of cases known, extreme caution is still strongly advised. High-risk groups include intravenous drug users, kidney dialysis patients, healthcare professionals, persons with multiple sex partners, recipients of blood transfusions before July 1992, and infants born to infected mothers. It is believed that the risk of neonatal transfer of the hepatitis C virus increases if the mother is infected with HIV. The incubation period for hepatitis C is usually six to nine weeks. The infected person may feel a sudden onset of flu-like symptoms that seem to linger. Others may gradually develop symptoms over a long period of time. Symptoms may include fatigue, low-grade fever, headache, sore throat, decreased appetite, nausea, vomiting, aching joints, dark urine, light stools, and pain in the right side over the area of the liver. In some cases, jaundice may appear. Hepatitis C is a progressive disease that can cause death due to liver failure or hepatocellular carcinoma (liver cancer).

HCV-related chronic liver disease may take up to 20 or more years to develop. It is now known that hepatitis B and HIV are often present in patients with HCV. Therefore, testing for each of these diseases is indicated. Screening for HCV is not routine. However, patients in high-risk categories should consider screening. These include the following:

- Those with a history of I.V. drug abuse

- Those with chronic hemodialysis

- Those with a history of a blood transfusion before June 1992

- Living in the same house as someone with HCV

- Sexual partners of someone with HCV who is in a nonmonogamous relationship

- History of sharing intranasal devices for drugs such as cocaine

- Those with a history of liver disease

- Healthcare providers who received a needle-stick injury from a person with HCV

Screening for contact with blood or body fluids from someone known to have the hepatitis C virus starts immediately after exposure. Testing is repeated in 4-6 months if the first test is negative. The HCV RNA test can be administered as early as 4-6 weeks.

Hepatitis D, also called delta hepatitis, is caused by a very small virus that cannot replicate on its own. Instead, it requires the presence of the hepatitis B virus. Hepatitis D can become chronic and is found only in patients with hepatitis B. It can cause a patient with a mild case of hepatitis B to develop a severe, chronic hepatitis and cirrhosis of the liver. It is estimated that hepatitis D is responsible for about 50% of fulminant hepatitis cases, which is a rare form of hepatitis that causes massive damage to the liver and eventually can lead to coma and death, possibly within two weeks. As the disease progresses, the patient may experience cerebral edema (swelling in the brain), brainstem compression, gastrointestinal bleeding, respiratory failure, cardiac failure, and kidney failure.

Hepatitis E is a virus transmitted through the fecal to oral route similar to hepatitis A. As in hepatitis A, it first enters the gastrointestinal tract, begins reproducing, and then spreads to the liver where it multiplies in the liver cells.

Hepatitis G is a virus transmitted through contaminated blood products. As in hepatitis B, C, and D, it enters the bloodstream, travels to the liver, and begins to reproduce. When the body's natural defenses attack the infected cells, the liver becomes inflamed.

Multiple Sclerosis

Multiple sclerosis (MS) is a debilitating disease affecting the brain and spinal cord. It is a major cause of disability in young adults, usually striking between the ages of 20 and 40. It is more common in women than in men.

There are five main types of MS, ranging from relatively mild symptoms that do not worsen and do not cause permanent disability to progressive deterioration without periods of remission. In a small number of MS patients, the disease progresses rapidly, sometimes causing complete disability and death within a few months of onset.

MS causes inflammation in portions of the nervous system that results in the destruction of the myelin sheaths that cover the nerve fibers. Areas of sclerosis or scarring remain that inhibit nerve signals. This can lead to visual impairment, muscle weakness, numbness, decreased coordination, paralysis, tremors, urinary and bowel incontinence, mood swings, and difficulty with speech. In advanced stages, patients can exhibit forgetfulness and confusion, sometimes referred to as "MS dementia."

As of this writing, the exact cause of MS is unknown, but a great deal of research has led to some possibilities—including a slow-acting viral infection and an auto-immune response of the nervous system, meaning the immune cells in one's body destroy the cells that produce myelin sheaths, or the nerve fiber covering. Diagnostic tests may include an electroencephalogram (EEG), a lumbar puncture, psychological testing, and a CT scan.

Parkinson's Disease

Parkinson's disease is a slow-progressing neurological disease. On average, deterioration progresses over a period of about ten years. Men are affected more often than women. Onset usually occurs in middle age or older, but may also occur at a younger age. It is believed that the cause of this illness is a deficiency in dopamine which prevents brain cells from performing their normal function within the central nervous system. Death usually occurs from aspiration pneumonia or another type of infection.

In general, symptoms progress to muscle rigidity; cramping in the neck, trunk, and legs; tremors; difficulty walking, with frequent falls; a high-pitched monotone voice; flat affect (lack of facial expression); body bent forward; difficulty swallowing; and eyes fixed upward.

Much research is being done to discover a cure for Parkinson's disease, but at present none exists. Treatment involves replacement medication for decreased dopamine levels. Often this decreases the severity of symptoms. Physical therapy is also used to help maintain normal muscle tone. In some cases, patients may opt for neurosurgery, but this is usually more of an option when the patient is comparatively young and otherwise healthy. Surgery is not a cure and is performed for palliative reasons to help relieve symptoms. A great deal of spiritual and emotional support is needed for patients with this cruel and debilitating illness.

In conclusion, I hope this chapter has provided you with enough information to serve as a starting point from which you can build more detailed knowledge on the subject of concern.

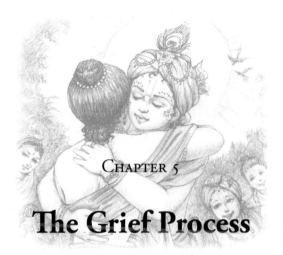

Chapter 5

The Grief Process

The time between diagnosis of a terminal illness and passing away can be filled with significant emotional and spiritual growth—not only for the patient, but for the caregiver and family members as well. It would be a remarkable achievement if the sense of peace that seems to come with accepting the eventuality of one's death, or that of a loved one, could be easily gained without a great amount of endeavor. Unfortunately, this is not always the case.

For the patient, coming to terms with imminent death may cause such crippling anxiety that everyday stressors may appear insurmountable. The tension is not exclusive to the patient, but can also be experienced by the caregiver and other family members who may be battling with their own feelings of guilt, anger, resentment, and fear. If you as the caregiver are tired—even exhausted—these feelings may not be easily resolved and could lead to overwhelming emotional turmoil. Anyone involved in a hospice situation is encouraged to come to terms with inner conflicts. It also becomes necessary to resolve unsettled conflicts between one another. This internal and external "mending" leads to an appreciation of each other's association and of the limited time you have with one another. This becomes especially important for devotees.

Fortunately, as Vaishnavas we have a wealth of spiritual knowledge available to assist in our transcendence of material hardships. But each of us walks alone on our spiritual journey and each of us varies in our needs. For some, caring for a dying loved one and preparing for the inevitable loss of that devotee may create more emotional turbulence than for others. Generally, it is helpful to clear away emotional pain that may create obstacles in spiritual life. It has been the experience of many senior Vaishnavas in our Krishna consciousness movement that unsettled emotional conflict often surfaces, requiring resolution years later. For this reason, I have included this chapter in order to provide an understanding of what the terminally-ill patient may be experiencing on an emotional level, as well as to assist you, the caregiver, in your emotional and spiritual growth at a time when your strength may often be tested.

As previously described, grief often begins for the patient at the time of diagnosis. Similarly, caregivers and family members may begin the grief process at this time as well. In fact, anyone who has a relationship with the patient and who will feel a sense of loss by his passing away will experience grief on some level. Just as Krishna consciousness is a process with necessary steps required to achieve greater understanding, grief is also thought of as a process leading to acceptance of one's own death or the eventual death of someone close to us. This concept, involving various stages of dying, has been written about at great length by Elisabeth Kubler-Ross, MD, who began her pioneering work with terminally-ill patients many years ago. Dr. Kubler-Ross spent decades caring for the dying, young and old, and found a common thread of emotional thought experienced by those facing imminent death. Similar grief reactions can be seen not only in the dying, but also in those experiencing a traumatic life event, such as a divorce or any life-altering occurrence where great loss is felt.

As described by Kubler-Ross, the stages of grief are: denial, anger, bargaining, depression, and acceptance.

It is important to note that not every terminally-ill patient experiences all of these stages or goes through them in the expected order. For example, I have seen patients who were passive by nature and had strong religious beliefs. Therefore they never felt angry when told they had less than six months to live. Other patients felt depressed one day and angry the next. These stages are not carved in stone and certainly a person who is dying has the right to react in his or her own unique way.

Similarly caregivers, family members, and close friends may experience these stages of grief according to their individuality. Sometimes the patient may reach the stage of acceptance while a family member struggles with anger. For example, I once had a 76-year-old patient who had worked hard to accept his imminent death after suffering from congestive heart failure. This strong and caring man, who was a Baptist minister, then spent his final days trying to console his adult children who, unfortunately remained angry even after his death.

The following is a discussion of each of the five stages of grief in the order in which they are generally thought to occur.

Denial

When someone is told that she has a terminal illness, the initial reaction is often one of denial. Many times, it is the reaction of loved ones as well. Denial is used as a coping mechanism to shield one from life-altering news that appears overwhelming. It is normal and is simply a way of adjusting. Remind yourself that adjustment takes time.

A newly-diagnosed patient may avoid speaking to anyone about his illness or may even avoid contact with friends or family members for fear they may mention his disease. Often a patient blames the doctor or claims the test results were false. It is common for a patient in denial to continue talking about the future and make plans for a time span that is well beyond his prognosis.

An example of this occurred when my mother-in-law was dying of metastatic breast cancer. She ordered a set of coins that were to arrive in the mail each month for one year. Obviously, she was not going to live long enough to receive the full set of coins, but her denial concerning the extent of her cancer greatly influenced her actions. Eventually, when her condition worsened, her strong religious beliefs helped her to accept the inevitable and she became very peaceful with her situation. Even after she accepted her fate, however, there were a few family members who remained in denial about her condition. They refused to plan for future round-the-clock care, stating, "We don't need to talk about that now because she won't be needing round-the-clock care for a long time." Statements like this are common when family members are having a difficult time accepting the reality of the situation. My experience with hospice families has been that, in general, if they have always lived with a "Let's not talk about it" policy, this attitude will persist even when a family member is terminally ill.

Denial acts as a type of barrier that keeps someone safe from the shocking reality of impending death. Well-meaning friends and family members may think it is beneficial to encourage the patient to "face reality."

But it is unkind to push someone into facing such harsh news before he or she is ready. Dr. Kubler-Ross recommends that a patient's questions be answered honestly but that we should not volunteer information for which the patient has not yet asked, because he is probably not ready to hear it. A terminally ill patient will gradually feel loss on many levels, including loss of physical abilities and the independence to perform even the most minimal of tasks. The dying person also feels the loss of a lifetime of plans and expectations. Dr. Peter Kaye powerfully makes this point when he states, "Giving up hopes and dreams for the future can be more difficult than giving up objects which actually exist."

As devotees, we may be anxious for the patient to quickly accept her terminal condition so she can get on with the business of spiritually preparing for death. But for the caregiver, patience is once again required at this time.

Continued denial, however, can eventually become inappropriate and detrimental to one who is facing imminent death. Denial becomes inappropriate if it does not assist in the patient's adaptation to his illness or when it hinders other adjustments, such as practical, financial, emotional, and spiritual alterations. Its persistence becomes harmful when it causes additional anguish to the patient, family, and caregiver. It can also cause harm when it keeps the patient from accepting palliative treatment, such as pain medication. Trust your instincts and you will know when your patient's denial has extended to an inappropriate length of time.

Talking to a patient or loved one who is in denial about approaching death must be done delicately and with kindness. To test the extent of a patient's denial, ask, "Can you tell me what the doctor said about your illness?" This same question can be adjusted to test the denial of a loved one. Remember that there are many intricate layers to someone's denial. Each covering must be gently lifted with care. However, this does not mean that you offer false hope of recovery. If a patient is deceived in this way, he may lose trust in his caregivers when he feels himself growing weaker. It may also prevent him from settling any unfinished business. This stage is not an easy time for the caregiver. There is a very thin line between gently uncovering someone's denial and misleading him. I always found it helpful to tell my patients at this stage, "Of course, the Lord can always intervene but at this point your medical reports show you have a very serious illness." In this way, I never completely took away their hope, which is something Dr. Kubler-Ross suggests, but I never misled them either.

It should be noted that a patient often exhibits what has been termed "intellectualizing," which is the ability of the patient to describe the technical aspects surrounding his illness while not yet connecting to it on an emotional level. For example, she might be able to explain to her spouse that her cancer has metastasized to the liver, lungs, and bone. In fact, she may verbalize this in a matter-of-fact manner and appear to those around her to have accepted her prognosis. Still, this individual remains in denial. As a caregiver, support the patient and assist her in understanding her fate on an emotional level, so her grief work can begin.

If you are receiving assistance from a hospice agency, ask your hospice nurse to step in if prolonged denial becomes a problem in any way, either with the patient or family members. An experienced hospice nurse should be able to confront those involved so that hospice care, and the comfort of the patient, is not hindered. In time, most patients reach a point where denial no longer rescues them and speaking about their fears offers a sense of relief.

Anger

A person often moves from the denial stage to the anger stage, but again, this is not always the case. Of all the stages in the grief process, anger can be the most difficult to cope with, both for the person feeling angry and those who are the recipients of that anger. A patient may become angry when he or she realizes that death is nearing; family members or close friends may become angry when they realize that someone dear to them will soon be gone. Because of this, anger can create a disturbance in one's support system by alienating family and friends.

It is not unusual for a terminal illness to create a restructuring of family members and a change in roles. Time previously spent between some family members may lessen while others may spend more time together caring for and visiting with the ill patient. While good communication helps all concerned to adjust to these changes, anger weakens healthy communication between loved ones.

For the patient, the anger phase may be a time of asking questions such as "Why me?" or "Why has the Lord done this to me?" Anger may also be a way of masking fear. As a caregiver who spends much of your time with the patient, you will naturally be the recipient of much of this anger. In turn, this may cause anger in you, as you feel you are unappreciated and being treated unfairly. If this occurs, remind yourself that the patient is not angry with you but at the situation. The patient is becoming more dependent on you and others as each day passes. This sense of helplessness may feel unbearable at times and may exhibit itself through angry outbursts. Remind yourself that these outbursts are a sign of the patient going through the grief process. Try to imagine how you would react in a similar situation. It is especially important at this stage that you, the caregiver, receive assistance from others who can allow you to step out of the situation for a short time, collect your thoughts, and then return to your caregiver responsibilities more refreshed.

Bargaining

Typically, the next stage in the grief process is when one makes promises or attempts to enter into an agreement of some kind in order to prolong life. In a sense, the terminally ill patient now negotiates for more time. Promises are often made to the Lord, especially when a patient feels he has not lived up to the spiritual standards that were expected of him. For instance, the patient may pray, "If you allow me to live longer, I'll spend more time reading the scriptures." Not only will someone make promises to the Lord, but may pledge to family members to change bad habits in his life in the hope of prolonging his life. He may try to mend a damaged relationship, thinking God will be pleased and grant his desire to live longer. The bargaining stage of grief is a most unfortunate phase for the patient and is painful for the caregiver to watch. As with the other stages, loved ones may also experience a type of bargaining, thinking it may allow them more time with the patient. As a caregiver, encourage the patient or loved one to verbalize his or her feelings. Bargaining is often associated with guilt. If the object of guilt is communicated and dealt with, it may help to resolve this stage more easily. Once again, good communication is required to decrease anxiety for all concerned.

Depression

After the bargaining stage, a terminally-ill patient (as well as family members) may become depressed. Depression is the beginning of realizing that death will soon occur. For the patient, this usually arises when symptoms worsen. She becomes weaker and is more dependent on others. This is the time she may experience a tremendous sense of loss, as her independence decreases. As with the other stages of grief, a change in family roles plays a key part in depression, as well as the absence of a job or a particular devotional service that the patient was attached to performing. Beyond feeling "reactionary depression" because of these types of losses, a person experiences what is referred to as "preparatory depression" as she realizes impending death is near.

Sometimes it is difficult to distinguish between a depressed patient and one experiencing an advanced illness, because many of the signs of depression—such as difficulty sleeping, decreased appetite, weakness, and fatigue—are seen in both situations. If the person has a previous medical history of depression, it is not uncommon for him to experience it in the terminal stage. Yet even when the person does not have a history of depression, he may still become depressed at this stage of his grief work. Surprisingly, comments about suicide are not necessarily a sign of depression in a dying patient. They may simply be a way of communicating to others the severe emotional anguish he is experiencing. It may also be an attempt to retain some type of control in his life. However, any comment pertaining to taking his own life should be immediately brought to the attention of the family and hospice staff. In any case, sadness for some time is a natural part of dying for the conditioned soul and may be necessary in order to reach the stage of acceptance. Once again, a caregiver's listening skills and empathy are required. Often, though, this stage of grief is a quiet one. Someone who is dying may simply need your silent, yet strong, presence as a source of comfort.

Acceptance

The final phase of the grief process is acceptance. It is a time of resolution and inner peace, both for the patient and family members experiencing it. The dying patient is now able to truly focus on the "self" and become detached from the worldly events surrounding her. Verbal communication will decrease. She may also exhibit detachment from loved ones. This is sometimes emotionally traumatic for those who cannot comprehend what the patient is experiencing. I have often explained to hospice families that, at this stage, it is as if the patient has one foot in this world and one foot in the next. After a great deal of work, she is finally ready to face death. I am always in awe upon observing a patient who has successfully achieved this state of awareness. For a Vaishnava, this is the most glorious of times because she has completed her grief work and is now free to fully concentrate on remembering the Lord.

At times, the patient may express a desire to be left alone. As a caregiver, we need to respect and facilitate the patient's need for solitude. These private moments become very precious to one who is facing death. As long as the patient is able to make his desires known, it is best to allow him choices. For the Vaishnava patient, ask if he would like to hear a *bhajan* tape or if someone can visit and quietly chant Hare Krishna or read aloud scripture. As the patient becomes more quiet and internal, the atmosphere in the room should reflect his consciousness. Lighting should be kept dim in the evening. Voices, chanting, and music should be soft and peaceful. One of the caregiver's duties at this time is to explain to loved ones that the patient's silence reflects tranquility and a sense of peace that comes with surrendering to the Lord's will. It is a time to rejoice for the Vaishnava who has come so far in preparing to die.

After discussing how we adults may experience the five stages of grief, we need to turn our attention to a much younger group, who may respond in a different manner to anticipatory grieving.

When Young Children are Involved

In general, Vaishnava children hear about death and dying from an early age because preparing one's consciousness for the time of death is an integral part of the Krishna consciousness philosophy. However, when a young child must watch someone die who is close to her, she will have her own understanding of the situation, depending on age, cognitive development, and emotional maturity level.

It is believed that infants also grieve. When someone has been consistently present in a baby's life, he will have a sense of something missing when that caregiver passes away. The baby will probably cry more, may have trouble sleeping, and at times may be inconsolable. Being held and cradled when a grieving baby cries will reassure him that he is still loved and safe.

Young children exhibit grief more through behavior than words. For example, a child who is easily upset may be feeling confused but simply lacks the words to verbalize his uncertainty. A child who is angry because of the patient's terminal condition might misbehave more frequently or argue with others. Watch for conduct that is out of character for that child as clues to deeper feelings. Also, for children, grief may be exhibited through play. Those around the child should be aware of "games" with themes surrounding death and immortality. Conversations children have while pretending to role-play may reveal hidden emotions. Artwork may also disclose thoughts and feelings that the child is unable to verbalize.

Children must be allowed to grieve in their own way and not have to conform to adult ideas concerning grief. Allow the child opportunities to ask questions about the terminal condition of the patient. Young children often think that someone's illness and ensuing death may be their fault. They may harbor feelings of guilt and require reassurance that they did not cause the situation. Krishna consciousness assists those of all ages to transcend material grief, but a grieving child requires an enormous amount of emotional sensitivity on our part so unresolved issues do not surface in adulthood.

Young children often find it easier to discuss disturbing events when they are physically engaged in other activities, such as playing with toys or dolls, and not looking directly at the adult who is speaking with them. For instance, you may find an opportune moment to discuss concerns about a loved one's illness while the child is drawing or coloring. If the child has a bedtime ritual such as storytelling or discussing the day's events, he or she may feel secure at this time and more willing to share thoughts and feelings.

Since the developmental stage of a child affects his or her concept of death, I have included the following brief summaries of various age groups, their cognitive understanding of death, and possible signs of distress.

- **Ages 2-4** – Children at this age are self-centered and literally think that the world revolves around them. This is the preconceptual stage when they are unable to grasp concepts. Death is seen as abandonment, reversible, and nonpermanent. Anxieties may exhibit themselves through regression of certain behaviors, such as wanting to be fed, asking to drink from a bottle instead of a cup, and bed-wetting.

- **Ages 5-7** – Children at this age are gaining more independence while exploring the world outside of the self. They are expanding their use of language. They tend to ask many "Why?" questions. Children at this age may feel guilty because they link thoughts with events. For example, if the child was once angry and wished harm on the loved one who is now terminally ill, he may feel responsible for causing the patient's disease. This is a time when fantasy is believed to be true. Death is still seen as reversible. Anxieties may be revealed through role-play. Children at this age may experience nightmares and be more violent in their play.

- **Ages 8-11** – Children at this age are entering the beginning of logical thinking. Death is seen as a punishment. They are beginning to see death as irreversible and final. Anxieties may cause problems with concentration in school. They may isolate themselves from others. They may experience disturbances with sleep. They may worry about how life will change after the death of a loved one. For example, they may become overly concerned about having to move to a new home or even to a new city, leaving behind family and friends. These adjustments become secondary losses to the already traumatic event of losing someone dear to them.

- **Ages 12-18** – This age group can now problem solve and is capable of abstract thinking. They are capable of conceptualizing death and to make sense of it on their own terms in combination with what they have been taught throughout childhood. Anxieties can manifest through depression and anger. Adolescents may isolate themselves while at home, spending more time in their bedroom. It is sometimes easier for children at this age to talk about the situation to those outside the family.

It is important to note that children grieve in cycles throughout childhood. In fact, their grief work may continue throughout life. At each new level of development throughout childhood and adolescence, they re-process past significant events through the lens of newly-acquired maturity and cognitive abilities. For example, a baby who loses a parent may re-experience his grief when he begins to develop language skills and can verbalize his feelings of loss. When reaching adolescence, he may process the loss again using his newly-developed capacity for abstract thinking. Important milestones in life will cause the sense of loss to resurface. Birthdays, graduations, weddings and other rites of passage are sad reminders of his missing loved one.

The Role of the Caregiver

For adults and children alike, a terminal illness creates an upheaval for all concerned. It is often the caregiver who bears the weight of that turbulence. You may find yourself going from the patient's room to the living room, only to become aware of family members who need your strength and guidance just as much as the patient will. As a caregiver, gather your emotional and spiritual strength so you can be a source of strength and comfort to those around you. However, in the midst of holding up everyone else, do not neglect your own sense of loss. You have the right to grieve in your own unique way as well.

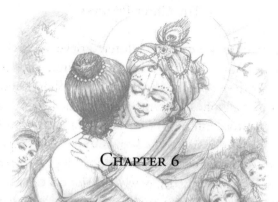

CHAPTER 6

Pain Management and the Use of Allopathic Medicine

The fundamental understanding when assessing pain is to accept that the patient's self-report is the most reliable indicator of the intensity of his own pain. According to Margo McCaffery, RN, MS, and pain management specialist, "Pain is whatever the experiencing person says it is, existing whenever he says it does."

Pain is subjective, influenced by one's childhood, life experiences, and culture. A patient's perception and reaction to pain is also influenced by mood, morale, and pain threshold. Therefore, observations of a patient's behavior should never override what the patient is describing. Similarly, sleep or sedation should never be mistaken for pain relief. Someone with severe pain can fall asleep simply from exhaustion, but may later awaken in agony.

Some patients hesitate to admit they are in pain or even deny they are experiencing pain at all. This can occur for many reasons. Some terminally ill patients fear they will become addicted to pain medicine if taken on a regular basis. (Family members often believe this as well and reinforce the patient's beliefs.) Some fear the side effects associated with pain medications. Others see it as a weakness to admit they are in pain, or simply feel they will become a burden to the caregiver if they complain. In addition, some patients fear they will not be alert and clear-thinking if they succumb to taking medicines for pain. Pain medications, if given correctly, can give the suffering patient relief without the side effect of extreme sedation. There is a saying among hospice professionals regarding pain management, "Start low; go slow." This is discussed in more depth throughout this chapter.

Whatever the reason, the caregiver should encourage the patient to verbalize her discomfort in order to achieve relief. As the caregiver, reassure the patient that medication correctly taken for pain relief is rarely psychologically addicting and that any possible side effects, such as nausea or constipation, can usually be relieved. Explain to your patient that complaints of pain will never be seen as troublesome or as a sign of weakness. Tell him that you are there to ease his discomfort in any way possible. Inevitably a patient's condition will worsen, making it difficult or even impossible for him to verbalize his pain. The caregiver should assume that if the patient's disease caused pain when he was alert, then his disease process is still causing pain even though he is unable to express it. At this point, a caregiver should watch for subtle signs of pain, such as frowning, facial grimacing (especially when being repositioned), moaning, and rapid breathing and heartbeat. Even when these signs are not present, pain medications should be continued round the clock to achieve a therapeutic blood level for comfort. This will ensure that a patient's final days are as peaceful and pain-free as possible.

Pain Assessment

When assessing a patient's pain, hospice staff will often consider its location, onset, character, intensity, frequency, and duration. A terminally ill patient will often have different types of pain in several locations. However, not all complaints of pain may be disease-related. For example, a patient might complain of general soreness that may be caused from being bedridden and immobile. To accurately assess a patient's pain, it is best to ask the following questions:

- Where is the pain?

- When did it start?

- What type of pain is it? Is it dull, throbbing, stabbing, aching, or burning? (This will give clues as to the source of the pain, such as bone, visceral, nerve, or muscle. For example, nerve pain tends to feel like an intense burning or tingling pain, while bone pain may feel like a throbbing or aching pain. Allow the patient to describe the pain in his own words.)

- What is the intensity of the pain? Is it mild, discomforting, distressing, excruciating? A commonly used pain rating scale is the 0-10 pain scale. You can implement the 0-10 pain scale by first explaining that zero means no pain and 10 is the most unbearable pain ever experienced. Ask the patient to rate her pain between 0 and 10. Visualization of the pain scale sometimes assists the patient to better assess her degree of discomfort. You can make a 0-10 pain-rating scale by drawing a horizontal line on a piece of paper. Write a zero on one end and a 10 on the opposite end. Fill in the numbers in between. The 1-4 range is considered to be mild pain, the 5-6 range is moderate pain, and the 7-10 range is severe pain. However, one patient may be able to tolerate pain in the 6 or 7 range, for example, while another patient may need pain relieved to a 1 or 2 in order to be comfortable. Again, pain is subjective and individualized.

- How long does the pain last? Is it sporadic? Is it constant?

- Does the pain feel worse at a specific time of day?

- What makes the pain worse? Sitting? Standing? Walking?

- Does anything help to relieve the pain?

- Has there been a change in the pain since yesterday or this morning?

Although it is the goal, zero pain relief is not always possible with a terminal illness. McCaffery suggests, "Satisfactory pain relief is a level of pain that is noticeable, but not distressing, and one that enables the patient to sleep, eat, and perform other required or desired physical activities."

Constant reassessment of the patient's pain is essential. Terminal pain can intensify and new pain can develop, sometimes daily. Inappropriate assessment of a patient's pain can result in ineffective treatment and unnecessary suffering.

A Word about Choices

Some patients may desire a more alternative approach to their pain management rather than agree to the use of allopathic medicine. However, having been trained as a nurse in a more conventional setting in the West, my education and expertise in pain management involves allopathic medications. I have seen them work. I have seen that when given correctly they diminish excruciating pain in patients about to die, making their last days comfortable ones. I have also seen a few patients experience intolerable side effects to these same medications. Most of the common side effects that can occur with the use of allopathic pain medicine can be easily controlled. Certainly the reader is invited to explore other types of therapies for pain management. However, it is never recommended to administer medicine of any kind without the proper guidance of a healthcare professional. The patient's physician, as well as any hospice staff involved in the patient's care, should be consulted before trying any alternative or over-the-counter medication. (Even some herbs can have adverse effects, especially when taken with certain medications.) The main concern should be keeping your patient as pain-free as possible with as few side effects as possible. (Chapter 9 addresses complementary therapies that may be helpful for symptom management in a hospice setting.)

Most hospices in the West have guidelines similar to the pain-management principles stated in this chapter. Even when a patient is receiving hospice care, however, he has the right to refuse a medication and/or discuss any apprehension related to the medications recommended by the hospice staff.

Three Major Analgesic Groups—
Non-opioid, Opioid, and Co-analgesics

Non-opioids

In general, non-opioid medications consist of acetaminophen, aspirin, and non-steroidal anti-inflammatory drugs (NSAIDs). NSAIDs work on the peripheral nervous system, the portion of the nervous system outside the central nervous system which consists of the brain and spinal cord. They work at the site of injury and are usually given for mild pain, as an anti-inflammatory, or as an antipyretic (fever reducer). Many non-opioids can be purchased over the counter without a prescription, such as acetaminophen (e.g., Tylenol), aspirin, ibuprofen (e.g., Advil, Motrin, or Nuprin), and naproxen sodium (e.g., Aleve). Acetaminophen is also known as paracetamol in some countries. Examples of NSAIDs requiring a physician's prescription include ketorolac tromethamine (Toradol), indomethacin (Indocin), nabumetone (Relafen), and choline magnesium trisalicylate (Trilisate). As with most medication, NSAIDs have a ceiling dose when used daily. Do not take more of this medication than is recommended. An overdose of ibuprofen can cause damage to your stomach or intestines. The maximum amount of ibuprofen usually recommended for adults is 800 mg per dose or 3200 mg per day (4 maximum doses within 24 hours). Use only the smallest amount of ibuprofen needed to get relief from your pain, swelling, or fever. Over-the-counter tablets of ibuprofen generally contain 200 mg, but a prescription dose can contain up to 800 mg per tablet. This medication should never be taken on an empty stomach. It is recommended that ibuprofen be taken with food or milk to prevent stomach upset. Therefore, to avoid toxicity it is necessary to keep careful records of when and how much of the medication is given. Possible side effects of ibuprofen, as well as some other NSAIDs include, but are not limited to, dizziness, headache, nervousness, peripheral edema (swelling in the limbs), tinnitus (ringing in one or both ears), epigastric distress, nausea, stomach ulcers, diarrhea, constipation, prolonged bleeding time, itching, and rash. Acute renal failure is less common, but can be a life-threatening side effect. NSAIDs should always be taken with food and never on an empty stomach. Over-the-counter NSAIDs should never be administered to a patient without consulting a physician or hospice nurse because of possible adverse interactions with other medications. In addition, if one NSAID is ineffective in treating a patient's discomfort, trying another type of NSAID may prove to be more effective.

Aspirin, although an excellent analgesic for mild pain, has a high incidence of stomach irritation. It should always be taken with milk, food, a large glass of water, or an antacid to reduce gastrointestinal distress. It also works as an anti-inflammatory agent and as an antipyretic. Aspirin has a blood-thinning effect, and many cardiac patients take aspirin in small daily doses for its anticlotting factors. However, it is usually not recommended for a patient who is already taking a blood-thinning medication or to a patient with impaired kidney or liver function, a history of gastric ulcers, or other bleeding disorders. Enteric-coated aspirin is less likely to cause gastrointestinal discomfort, but since enteric-coated (as well as sustained-release) tablets are more slowly absorbed, it is not suitable for fast relief of pain, fever, or inflammation. As with NSAIDs, it is best to consult your physician or hospice nurse before administering over-the-counter aspirin, since it does not interact well with many prescription and nonprescription medications. When using enteric-coated aspirin, it should never be broken, crushed, or chewed.

Acetaminophen (e.g., Tylenol) tends to be milder on the stomach than aspirin or other NSAIDS but does not have the same anti-inflammatory effects. It is generally given for mild pain and to reduce fever. When a hospice patient is no longer able to swallow whole pills, acetaminophen may be given in other forms, such as liquid, chewable, or rectal suppositories. Acetaminophen suppositories often are used when a terminally ill patient is unresponsive, unable to swallow any form of medications, and needs relief from a fever. Side effects of acetaminophen are fewer than with NSAIDs and aspirin but can include rash, jaundice, and liver damage (from toxic doses). In a patient whose blood glucose levels are being monitored with a home monitoring system, acetaminophen can sometimes produce false-positive decreases in blood glucose levels. Generally, when used as a long-term therapy, acetaminophen dosage should not exceed 2000 mg daily, or the patient will run the risk of toxicity.

Opioids

Opioid is the preferred term to use for narcotic medication. Opioids are non-opium-derived synthetic drugs used for moderate to severe pain. Opioids work by attaching themselves to specific opiate receptors on cells in the central nervous system (brain and spinal cord). An important intervention in pain management (from mild to severe pain) is to anticipate and prevent pain rather than treating it as it occurs. Waiting for pain to reappear before administering the next dose of pain medication is futile and only serves to place the patient in a never-ending cycle of anguish and relief. This is why it is so important to administer round-the-clock dosages (i.e., given at set times throughout the day). No one should have to wait until he is writhing in pain before receiving medication for relief. Once pain occurs, it is more difficult to control. Anticipation on the part of the caregiver is the key to successful pain management. A patient's suffering only heightens when combined with the anxious expectation of oncoming pain. Once the patient's pain is controlled using a round-the-clock administration method, she becomes pain free (or as close to pain free as possible). She is then maintained on a steady dose of medication until the disease process exacerbates and the dose must again be increased for comfort.

Weak to Moderate Opioids

Some opioids are effective for mild to moderate pain, such as oxycodone (e.g., Percocet) or hydrocodone (e.g., Lortab or Vicodin). Many of these medications come in combination form and may contain acetaminophen or aspirin. Percocet, for example, contains acetaminophen. In many cases the acetaminophen or aspirin helps to give greater pain relief than if the opioid were used alone, but even in combination these weaker opioids have less analgesic effect than morphine or other more potent opioids. Care must be taken not to exceed the prescribed dose of these combination medicines, not only for the detrimental effects of receiving too much of the opioid, but because toxic levels of acetaminophen and aspirin can be equally dangerous.

Side effects of opioids vary according to the specific medication, but some adverse effects of these weak to intermediate medications may include, but are not limited to, dizziness, sedation, nausea, vomiting, constipation, rash, itching, headache, dry mouth, abdominal discomfort, and respiratory depression. The goal of using any opioid is for the patient to be as pain free as possible without sedation. The patient should be able to relate to his environment without feeling euphoric. Because nausea and constipation are common side effects of opioids, it is suggested that whenever any type of opioid is started, a laxative/stool softener such as senna (e.g., Senokot) or docusate sodium (e.g., Colace) be given regularly to avoid constipation. (Never wait until the patient is constipated to begin use of a laxative/stool softener.) Along with a laxative/stool softener, an antiemetic medication should be given on an "as needed" basis for nausea. It is recommended to have on hand an antiemetic that comes in suppository form in case the patient cannot tolerate it in pill form.

As of November 2010, the U.S. Food and Drug Administration (FDA) asked the pharmaceutical company that makes the prescription pain medications Darvon (generic name propoxyphene) and Darvocet/Darvocet-N (propoxyphene with acetaminophen) to withdraw the drugs from the U.S. market. The FDA says the drug propoxyphene puts patients at risk of potentially serious or fatal heart rhythm abnormalities. The medication is usually given for mild to moderate pain.

The director of the FDA's Office of Surveillance and Epidemiology stated, "We recommend to physicians (to) stop prescribing the drugs. As for patients, do not stop taking it, but we urge you to contact your health care professional. Do not delay. The drug's effectiveness in reducing pain is no longer enough to outweigh the drug's serious potential heart risks."

Commonly used opioids for mild to moderate pain include:

- **Lortab 7.5/500** (Lortab also comes in various strengths. The first number, 7.5, is the mg amount of hydrocodone bitartrate in each tablet. The second number, 500, is the mg amount of acetaminophen in each tablet.)

- **Percocet** (Contains 325 mg of acetaminophen and 5 mg of oxycodone hydrochloride.)

- **Percodan** (Contains 325 mg of aspirin and 5 mg of oxycodone hydrochloride.)

- **Roxicet 5/500** (Contains 500 mg of acetaminophen and 5 mg of oxycodone hydrochloride.)

- **Tylenol with Codeine** (This combination comes in numbers 1-4. All contain 300 mg of Tylenol with various doses of codeine ranging from 7.5 mg to 60 mg per tablet.)

- **Tylox** (Contains 500 mg of acetaminophen and 5 mg of oxycodone hydrochloride.)

- **Vicodin** (Contains 500 mg of acetaminophen and 5 mg of hydrocodone bitartrate.)

- **Vicodin ES** (Contains 750 mg of acetaminophen and 7.5 mg of hydrocodone bitrartrate.)

As you can see, it is essential to know the amount of aspirin or acetaminophen contained within each tablet of a combination medication to prevent a toxic level from accumulating with long-term use. If a weak to intermediate opioid is being used that contains aspirin and the patient is experiencing abdominal discomfort, notify the hospice nurse or the patient's physician. He or she may want the patient to switch to an opioid that contains acetaminophen which, in general, does not cause the same abdominal distress.

A commonly used extended-release medication, Oxycontin (oxycodone HCL), has the same analgesic ingredient as Percocet or Percodan, but does not contain acetaminophen or aspirin. Generally, Oxycontin is used to relieve moderate to severe pain. The tablet is administered orally every 12 hours with analgesic onset usually occurring within one hour. Side effects of oxycodone may include respiratory depression, constipation, nausea, vomiting, sedation, itching, headache, dry mouth, and dizziness. **Never break, crush, cut, or have the patient chew this medication or any other extended-release medicine.** This could lead to the rapid release of a potentially dangerous dose of oxycodone.

Strong Opioids

Strong opioids are suggested for most cancer-related and other moderate to severe pain. Some commonly-prescribed opioids used in hospice care include morphine sulfate, hydromorphone (Dilaudid), and Fentanyl.

Morphine Sulfate

Soft tissue and visceral pain (pain derived from internal organs) usually respond well to morphine sulfate, which comes in various forms and strengths and can be administered by various routes. In hospice care the oral route is preferred but is not always possible, as the patient's disease may make swallowing difficult. Often the disease itself, such as esophageal cancer, makes it impossible for the patient to take oral medications. Some patients may simply dislike swallowing pills. Some types of morphine can be given rectally as a suppository or are available in concentrated liquid form and can be given under the tongue using a dropper. When a medication is administered under the tongue, it is referred to as the sublingual route.

In general, certain routes of administering morphine are used as a last resort in palliative care. These routes include intravenous or IV (an injection into a catheter that has been placed in a vein), and intramuscular (an injection into a muscle). IVs are considered invasive, may cause infections, or may simply become a source of discomfort for the patient. IVs also limit mobility, thus diminishing a patient's quality of life. Injections given intramuscularly on a regular basis are inconvenient and can be painful, especially if a terminally ill patient has become emaciated through illness and loss of appetite.

Whatever route is used, the goal of morphine is to reduce the patient's pain without causing drowsiness. If morphine has been successful in reducing the patient's pain but he becomes drowsy, the dose of morphine should be reduced **without compromising the patient's pain relief**. Continuous reassessment of the patient's pain is essential since some types of pain, such as bone and nerve pain, respond poorly or not at all to morphine. Morphine sulfate comes in shorter-acting, instant/immediate-release forms as well as extended-release forms that last 12 to 24 hours.

Dispelling the Myths

There are many fears that surround the use of morphine. Some physicians are resistant to start a terminally ill patient on this medication, fearing that as tolerance develops to the drug, higher doses will be needed with less effective pain control. I have had many patients be afraid to take morphine for fear of addiction. Family members often express a concern that morphine will cause the patient to experience respiratory failure.

Unfortunately, these myths sometimes lead to poor pain management in terminally ill patients. Correct use of morphine means that it is given for a type of pain that responds well to morphine, such as visceral and soft tissue pain, and that the dose is correctly titrated, meaning the patient begins with a low dose and then receives increasing dosages in proper increments until his pain is relieved. If the pain increases again, the dose of morphine increases. If titration is done correctly, the patient's pain should be relieved without causing drowsiness.

For reasons unknown, some patients may develop a tolerance to morphine when receiving it intravenously. This usually does not occur when morphine is administered by oral, rectal, sublingual, subcutaneous, or intramuscular routes and is given for soft tissue or visceral pain. Once a patient's pain is controlled, she can stay on that same dose of morphine for weeks or months without developing a tolerance. Problems arise when morphine is given for pain that does not respond to the drug such as bone pain, nerve pain, or gastric distention. The medication is then mistakenly increased again and again, thinking that increased doses will bring pain relief; but if the pain is not morphine-receptive, no amount of this opioid will bring relief.

In addition, the continuous use of oral morphine does not produce a euphoric effect when used correctly for pain relief. This holds true for respiratory depression as well. As long as morphine is titrated correctly, and the dose is reduced if the patient exhibits excessive drowsiness, there should be no fear of morphine causing a patient's respirations to cease.

Instant / Immediate Release Morphine

In hospice care, instant/immediate-release morphine is commonly used when first starting a patient on morphine. Instant/immediate release morphine generally takes effect within twenty minutes after administration and has an analgesic effect of about 2-4 hours. Once a patient's pain is controlled, the dose can be converted to extended-release morphine and given every 12 hours round the clock. In addition, they now make extended-release morphine that is taken once every 24 hours. Instant/immediate-release morphine can then be used for "breakthrough pain relief" on an as-needed basis, along with long-acting morphine as the main pain reliever. Examples of shorter-acting, instant/immediate-release morphine sulfate include:

- **Roxanol Concentrate** - This is a concentrated solution of morphine sulfate that starts to give pain relief within about 15 minutes after administration and has its peak effect in about 30 minutes. It has a bitter taste. If tolerated by the patient, a measured dose can be mixed with a very small amount of fruit juice (1-2 tablespoons) to make the taste more pleasant. This form of morphine is usually given by using a dropper. Place a few drops at a time under the patient's tongue or against the inside cheek of the mouth where it is absorbed through the mucosa without the patient having to swallow. In patients who are at the end stage of their disease process, even a few drops of liquid placed near the inside of the cheek or under the tongue may cause choking. If choking becomes excessive, the physician or hospice nurse may want to switch to morphine sulfate suppositories.

- **Morphine Sulfate Instant Release** (MSIR) - This form of morphine also comes in a concentrated solution, as well as capsules and small tablets. The instant-release capsules can be emptied and mixed with a very small amount of applesauce or pudding (1-2 tablespoons) if the patient has difficulty swallowing the medication whole. The instant-release pills can be crushed and mixed with applesauce or pudding as well, if not tolerated whole.

- **Morphine Sulfate Elixir** - This type of morphine comes in various flavors and strengths. This is not in concentrated form, so a larger amount of liquid must be swallowed by the patient with each dose.

- **Morphine Suppositories** - These are given rectally, usually when the patient is unable to tolerate anything by mouth. Onset of pain relief begins in about 20-60 minutes after administration and usually lasts about four hours or so. As with other types of morphine, suppositories also come in various doses.

Extended-Release Morphine Sulfate

Extended-release morphine sulfate is long-acting, with a duration of 12-24 hours. Some patients may require it every eight hours, but this is not usually the case. This is given round the clock for pain relief and is a vital component of the patient's pain management. Again, a round-the-clock regimen is the best way to manage severe, chronic pain. A commonly used type of extended-release morphine sulfate is MS Contin, which comes in various doses and can be given orally or rectally if the patient is unable to swallow tablets. **<u>Never crush, break, or cut extended-release morphine!</u>** The patient will receive the entire dose too quickly rather than receiving it in small increments over the appropriate time. This can cause serious side effects, including respiratory arrest. There are other sustained-release morphine sulfate tablets and capsules as well, made by various pharmaceutical companies. The tablets and capsules vary in size, dosage, and cost.

Adverse reactions to morphine sulfate (short- or long-acting) include, but are not limited to, sedation, euphoria, seizures, dizziness, nightmares (with long-acting oral forms), hallucinations, nervousness, depression, nausea, vomiting, constipation, urine retention, rash and itching, respiratory depression or arrest, and cardiac arrest.

Whenever opioid therapy of any kind is initiated, the patient will usually experience an increase in sedation lasting approximately 48-72 hours. This initial drowsiness is temporary, and the patient should become more alert as he or she adapts to the medication. It has been noted that many patients exhibit excessive sleep when starting an opioid because they have been coping with unrelieved pain for a long period of time. Pain relief will then provide total relaxation, with a subsequent undisturbed sleep that can replace weeks or months of agonizing exhaustion. However, a caregiver should always wake the patient to administer the next regularly-scheduled dose of pain medication. Otherwise, the patient may awaken in pain and his round-the-clock schedule will need to be adjusted. If the patient cannot be easily awakened when he was easily awakened prior to receiving medication, has unusually slow or shallow respirations (normal is 16-20 respirations per minute), is hallucinating when awake, or has abnormally slurred speech, the caregiver should call the hospice and report the symptoms to the nurse before administering the next prescribed dose of pain medication. If a terminally ill patient has been on a stable dose of opioids for several days or longer and then becomes weaker, less alert, has cool extremities, and decreased or erratic respirations, his disease process may be worsening and he is probably moving closer to death. Notify the hospice nurse as soon as these symptoms appear.

Dilaudid

Dilaudid (hydromorphone hydrochloride) comes in subcutaneous, intramuscular, and intravenous injections, tablets, suppositories, and syrup. In a hospice setting, it is usually given orally for moderate to severe pain. As with morphine, hydromorphone binds with opiate receptors in the central nervous system and alters the perception of and emotional response to pain. As with other pain medications, it should be administered before the patient has intense pain to produce a better analgesic effect. Pain relief can be felt about 30 minutes after taking this medication. It is a strong opioid but has a short duration of only about four hours, so patients may run the risk of suffering from a "roller coaster effect," that is, feeling pain, then four hours of relief, then experiencing the pain again. This is avoided by using an extended-release, longer-acting pain medication that is given on a regular basis before the pain returns. Side effects of hydromorphone may include, but are not limited to, sedation, dizziness, euphoria, hypotension (low blood pressure), nausea, vomiting, constipation, urine retention, and respiratory depression.

Subcutaneous Medication Infusion

Since the first edition of this book was published, many hospice agencies now use a subcutaneous infusion system for medication administration. Simply stated, this is the insertion of an intravenous (IV) catheter needle into the subcutaneous tissue rather than into a vein. Following the insertion of an IV catheter needle into the tissue site, the needle is then discarded and all that remains in place is the plastic cannula, or thin tube. This cannula can stay in place for up to seven days for either intermittent or continuous medication infusions, such as with morphine or methadone, for severe pain. This procedure is sometimes done with a metal butterfly needle rather than an IV catheter system, but the use of a butterfly needle requires site changes more often than when using an IV catheter.

Effective pain and symptom relief in the terminally ill patient is an important element of quality end-of-life care. In some individuals, the use of a subcutaneous site is required in order to reach this goal. This procedure reduces the number of injections the patient receives since the medication is injected directly into the tubing, which then enters the body's subcutaneous tissue, rather than having to subject a fragile patient to countless needle sticks.

Some common indications for the use of the subcutaneous route for medication administration include, but are not limited to:

- Conditions that would prevent the use of oral administration of medications such as dysphagia (difficulty swallowing) due to a variety of reasons

- Decreased level of consciousness toward the end of life

- Intestinal obstruction

- Nausea and vomiting

- Advanced dementia or agitated delirium

The injection site should be assessed frequently for signs and symptoms of infection, cannula misplacement, and overuse of site. This would include: leaking, redness, exudate, localized heat, localized inflammation, pain, tenderness, hardness, burning, swelling, scarring, itching, or bruising.

A Word about Using Demerol in Hospice Care

Meperidine hydrochloride (Demerol) is a synthetic opioid that comes in tablets, syrup, and injections. It has a rapid onset with lesser stigma attached to it than morphine, but is short-acting, lasting only one to three hours. It is highly irritating to the soft tissue and should never be given using continuous subcutaneous infusions. Meperidine hydrochloride is not recommended for hospice patients who suffer with chronic pain requiring long-term medication. Meperidine and its active metabolite, normeperidine, a central nervous system stimulant, accumulate in the body and can quickly reach toxic levels, especially in patients with impaired kidney function. Meperidine toxicity can appear in only a few days. Symptoms of toxicity include mild negative mood swings within 24 hours of receiving meperidine. This progresses to irritability, tremors, twitches, and seizures. It is not the drug of choice for a terminally ill patient.

Non-morphine Opioids

A common medication used for severe pain is Fentanyl Transdermal System (Duragesic Patch). Fentanyl also comes in intravenous and intramuscular injection forms, but in hospice, the transdermal patch is used more often. I have used the Fentanyl Patch many times with patients and have had good results, but, as with anything, it has its pros and cons. For a patient who cannot tolerate morphine sulfate, but still needs relief from severe pain, a Duragesic Patch may be appropriate and convenient. It is a small patch that comes in various dosages. The patch is simply placed on a fleshy, non-irritated, non-irradiated part of the body, such as the upper arm, flank, or thigh. Placing it over a bony prominence can inhibit absorption of the medication. The patch is then changed every three days (72 hours), although a small number of patients may require that it be changed every 48 hours. Either way, Fentanyl medication is slowly released from the patch, through the skin, and eventually into the bloodstream. It is noninvasive, painless, and often effective for pain relief. The patient may even shower or bathe with the patch on if it is secured with a clear bandage dressing. A Duragesic Patch may be appropriate for patients who have been unsuccessful with oral opioids, cannot tolerate morphine, or for patients who have their pain level stabilized. Patients with colon cancer may experience malabsorption of oral pain medications and may benefit from using a Duragesic Patch for pain relief. However, it is not recommended for patients who require frequent medication adjustment (titration). It is difficult to titrate the dose of medication using a Duragesic Patch because it may take up to six days for the patient to reach equilibrium on the new dose. Obviously, it is not the route to use when a patient is having a pain crisis and requires fast relief.

Serum drug levels rise for the first 24 hours after application of the patch, so pain relief cannot be evaluated on the first day of use. Your hospice nurse will probably provide a shorter-acting opioid to be given as needed for breakthrough pain relief while the patient is waiting for the full effects of the Duragesic Patch. When a Duragesic Patch is removed, approximately fifty percent of the drug remains in one's system for 17 hours. There are several pharmaceutical companies who make various types of short-acting Fentanyl medicine for "breakthrough pain relief" when the patient using the long-acting Fentanyl Duragesic patches suddenly experiences an exacerbation of pain that requires a short-acting, lower dose medicine that enters the bloodstream quickly when the patient needs to immediately address that sudden "burst of pain." One company produces a "lollipop-type," fast-acting Fentanyl that is much like sucking on a lollipop, but this medication gets dissolved quickly through the mucous membranes within the mouth. It comes in various doses and is titrated as needed. As with any breakthrough medication, if more and more doses are needed within a 24 hour period to relieve the patient's pain to a tolerable level, then the doctor should discuss the patient's options, such as increasing the main form of long-acting medication which in this case would be the Fentanyl Duragesic Patch. When the long-acting medication is increased, the breakthrough medication is always increased as well and is still prescribed on an as-needed basis with parameters such as "Every 2-4 hours as needed for breakthrough pain." You can see how important it is for the caregiver to keep an accurate record of when all medications are taken, including any breakthrough medicines so the hospice nurse and physician are aware of any need to titrate the medications as needed for the patient's comfort.

Co-analgesics

Co-analgesics, or adjuvant medications, are given to target specific types of pain. Many of these drugs have been used to treat other conditions prior to the discovery of their analgesic properties. For example, a patient with cancer may be receiving morphine for pain relief, but may still complain of nerve pain from compromised or damaged nerves. Therefore, a co-analgesic such as amitriptyline, a tricyclic antidepressant, is often given for relief of neuropathic discomfort.

Because morphine and other opioids do not relieve every type of pain, co-analgesics, often given with an opioid, can provide effective relief of pain that may not be experienced with the opioid alone. For example, even though morphine is the drug of choice for cancer pain, if a patient's cancer has metastasized to the bone, she may still require an NSAID to relieve her bone pain.

Commonly Used Co-analgesics and their Use in Hospice Care

For Nerve Pain:

Nerve pain can occur for many reasons, such as diabetic neuropathy, certain types of cancer involving malignant nerve infiltration, or herpetic neuralgia caused by shingles (herpes zoster). It can be described as stabbing, burning, shooting, or tingling ("pins and needles"). Nerve pain can be so severe that it interrupts sleep. In addition, patients with nerve pain often experience an increase in depression. Because nerve pain generally responds poorly to morphine, tricyclic antidepressants are often given to target this type of pain and not for their antidepressant effects. Analgesic benefits are not achieved immediately, but may take several days to 1-2 weeks to provide relief. In general, tricyclic antidepressants have many side effects such as dry mouth, constipation, and sedation, and therefore are not tolerated by everyone. If sedation becomes a problem, ask the hospice nurse or physician if the medication can be given at bedtime to minimize daytime side effects. Examples of tricyclic antidepressants used for nerve pain include:

- amitriptyline (Elavil)
- desipramine hydrochloride (Norpramin)
- nortriptyline hydrochloride (Pamelor)
- doxepin hydrochloride (Sinequan)
- imipramine hydrochloride (Tofranil)

Anticonvulsants may also be given as co-analgesics for some types of nerve pain. As with the tricyclic antidepressants, pain relief does not occur immediately. Side effects can include, but are not limited to, dizziness, drowsiness, nausea, and headache. If an increase in dosage is required to alleviate nerve pain, adverse reactions may be minimized if the dosage is increased gradually. Examples of anticonvulsants often used in hospice care to relieve nerve pain include:

- carbamazepine (Tegretol)
- clonazepam (Klonopin)
- gabapentin (Neurontin)
- phenytoin (Dilantin)

Corticosteroids have also been proven to reduce nerve pain in some patients. They are thought to be effective in reducing nerve compression. Examples of steroids used to relieve some types of nerve pain include:

- dexamethasone (Decadron)
- prednisone

As a co-analgesic, corticosteroids are useful in treating a variety of symptoms besides nerve compression pain. Some of the benefits derived from their use include improved appetite, improved mood and sense of well-being, reduced hypercalcemia (abnormally high calcium levels in blood), and reduced inflammation related to intra-cranial pressure sometimes caused by a brain tumor. Corticosteroids can relieve airway obstruction, decrease nausea, aid in relieving bowel obstruction, decrease pain from bone metastases, minimize side effects from radiation and chemotherapy, and bring relief from spinal cord compression. These drugs can also be administered for hepatomegaly (enlarged liver) and are useful for patients with head and neck tumors.

For Bone Pain:

Bone pain is often described as a dull, aching, or throbbing pain that is localized over a bony area and may worsen with movement. It is commonly associated with cancer that has metastasized to the bone. Breast, lung, and prostate cancer have a high rate of bone metastases but can occur with many other types of cancer as well. Typically, the earliest sites are the pelvis, ribs, and spine (usually the middle and lower spine).

Bone cancer causes pain that is thought by some to be the worst type of cancer-related pain. I once cared for a gentleman whose cancer had spread to his cervical spine (upper vertebra). Even the slightest adjustment of his pillow under his neck caused him to scream in agony. Another patient whose cancer had metastasized to his pelvis told me, "It feels like a knife is cutting through my bones."

Whenever possible, short-term, localized palliative radiation therapy is the treatment of choice for bone metastases. It can often provide pain relief by significantly reducing the size of the tumor. Many patients feel a decrease in pain within one to two weeks, but response time can take longer. When used for palliative reasons, radiation therapy is usually administered in relatively short courses, thus minimizing side effects. However, a patient may still experience nausea, vomiting, and skin irritation, including redness, soreness, and burning. Topical hydrocortisone cream can help reduce skin soreness. It is recommended that patients receiving radiation therapy avoid exposure to sunlight. Hair loss does not usually occur unless the head is irradiated.

If radiation therapy is not recommended or accepted by the patient, NSAIDs are the first drug of choice for bone pain because of their anti-inflammatory effects. Examples of NSAIDs commonly administered for bone pain include:

- naproxen sodium (Naprosyn)

- choline magnesium trisalicylate (Trilisate)

- ibuprofen (e.g., Motrin, usually 800 mg on a regular basis)

If bone pain persists after a trial use of NSAIDs, ask the physician or hospice nurse about using corticosteroids, such as prednisone or dexamethasone.

For Gastric Distention Pain:

Co-analgesics often given to relieve gastric distention are:

- metoclopramide hydrochloride (Reglan)

- simethicone (Gas-X, Mylanta, Phazyme)

For Rectal or Bladder Spasm Pain:

A co-analgesic often prescribed for this type of specific pain is hyoscyamine (e.g., Cystospaz, Levsin). However, for some patients a stronger medication may be required to relieve the severe spasms associated with certain types of cancer. One such combination medicine that comes in suppository form is made with belladonna, an anticholinergic, and opium. In general, neither of these medications are considered co-analgesics, but when combined can be effective in relieving severe spasm pain.

I once cared for a lovely elderly woman who suffered with unrelieved pain from bladder cancer. As her disease progressed, she attempted to jump out of her hospital bed in order to flee the painful bladder spasms she experienced day and night. No amount of morphine relieved her pain. When the hospice physician changed her medication to B&O suppositories (belladonna and opium), she was able to rest comfortably and lived out her final days with minimal discomfort.

Generally, morphine will not relieve pain caused by rectal or bladder spasms. Because B&O suppositories are not one of the more commonly prescribed medications, not every pharmacist will carry them. However, he or she may be able to special order them. **B&O suppositories are not recommended for children under the age of 12.**

For Muscle Spasm Pain:

The following co-analgesics may be helpful if your patient is experiencing pain from muscle spasms:

- diazepam (Valium)

- cyclobenzaprine hydrochloride (Flexeril)

The World Health Organization Three-Step Analgesic Ladder for Pain Control

The World Health Organization (WHO) provides a useful tool that illustrates the effective use of analgesic medications. On the first step of the ladder when a patient is experiencing mild pain, non-opioids are recommended, such as NSAIDs (e.g., Motrin, Naprosyn), acetaminophen (e.g., Tylenol), steroids, or aspirin. They can be given as needed when pain arises or on a round-the-clock basis. These non-opioids may be given with or without a co-analgesic, depending on the type of pain the patient is experiencing.

If pain persists or increases, the next step on the analgesic ladder is implemented by adding a weak to moderate opioid (e.g., Percocet, Tylenol #3, Vicodin). The weak to moderate opioid is usually given round the clock with a non-opioid to maintain a constant level of medication in the bloodstream so pain does not recur every few hours. On level two of the pain management ladder, a co-analgesic may or may not be used.

If pain persists or increases, pain management is advanced to the third level on the analgesic ladder by administering a stronger opioid (e.g., Morphine, Dilaudid, or Fentanyl patch). It may be given with or without a non-opioid, and with or without a co-analgesic. Adjustments are made according to the patient's needs.

In conclusion, a four-component medication system is generally used when treating severe chronic pain. This consists of:

1) An extended-release opioid given round the clock

2) An instant/immediate-release opioid given only as needed for "breakthrough pain"

3) A laxative/stool softener given regularly to avoid the side effect of constipation

4) An antiemetic to be used "as needed" for nausea.

Along with this four-component system, co-analgesics can be added to treat specific symptoms.

Pain management is one of the most important and satisfying duties of a caregiver. Regular communication with the patient as well as the hospice nurse is crucial in assuring optimum comfort. Each patient will have varied needs, but careful observation and constant reassessment on your part will greatly benefit your patient so his or her final days will be peaceful.

Commonly Used Medications in a Hospice Setting

Main Category	Sub Category	Example Medications	Uses	Possible Side Effects	Considerations Precautions
Non-Opioids	Non-Steroidal Anti-Inflamatory Drugs (NSAIDs)	Toradol Trilisate Relafen	Works on peripheral nervous system, at site of injury. Give for: mild pain, anti-inflamatory, fever reducer.	Dizziness, headache, nervousness, peripheral edema, tinnitus, nausea, stomach ulcers, diarrhea, constipation, prolonged bleeding time, itching and rash	* Acute renal failure can be a life-threatening side effect. Always take with food. * Do not exceed 1200 mg a day
	Aspirin		Mild pain, anti inflamatory fever reducer, blood thinner	Common adverse effect of aspirin is stomach irritation	Never give to a patient with impaired kidney or liver function, history of gastric ulcers, or other bleeding disorders. Give with milk, food or large glass of water.
	Acetaminophen	Tylenol	Mild pain, fever reducer	Rash, jaundice, liver damage (from toxic doses)	Comes in several forms (liquid, chewable, suppositories), can give false positive glucose results. * Do not exceed 2000 mg a day

Commonly Used Medications in a Hospice Setting

Main Category	Sub Category	Example Medications	Uses	Possible Side Effects	Considerations Precautions
Opioids	Weak to Moderate Opioid	Darvocet, Darvon, Lortab, Percocet, Percodan, Roxicet, Tylenol with codeine, Tylox, Vicodin	Works on the Central Nervous System (CNS). For mild to moderate pain	Dizziness, sedation, nausea, vomiting, constipation, rash, itching, headache, dry mouth, abdominal discomfort, respiratory depression	* Never exceed prescribed dose as this can lead to toxic levels of acetaminophen or asprin. Use with laxative/stool softener. Give an anti-emetic as needed for nausea (eg. Compazine or Tigan)
	Moderate to Strong Opioid	Oxycontin	Works on the Central Nervous System. For moderate to severe pain. Is extended release and is usually administered every 12 hours	Respiratory depression, nausea, vomiting, sedation, itching, headache, dry mouth, dizziness	Never break, crush, cut or chew. Best if given "round-the-clock". Use with laxative/stool softener. Give an anti-emetic as needed for nausea (eg. Compazine or Tigan).

Commonly Used Medications in a Hospice Setting

Main Category	Sub Category	Example Medications	Uses	Possible Side Effects	Considerations Precautions
Opioids	Strong Opioid	Morphine	For soft tissue and visceral pain. Severe chronic pain. Alters perception of and emotional response to pain.	Sedation, euphoria, seizures, dizziness, nightmares (with long acting oral forms), hallucinations, nervousness, depression, nausea, vomiting	Comes in oral, sublingual, suppository, IV, IM, or SQ injections. Doses need to be titrated. May cause sedation within the first 48-72 hours of use.
		Roxanol Concentrate		Constipation, urine retention, rash and itching, respiratory depression or arrest, cardiac arrest	Bitter taste, may mix with 1-2 tbsp. fruit juice. Place a few drops at a time under tongue or inside cheek.
		Morphine Sulphate Instant Release (MSIR)			Concentrated solution, capsules or small tablets. May mix capsules in 1-2 tbsp. applesauce or pudding.
		Morphine Sulphate Elixir			Not in concentrated form, so larger amount of liquid must be given.
		Morphine Suppositories			Use lubricant for comfort.

Commonly Used Medications in a Hospice Setting

Main Category	Sub Category	Example Medications	Uses	Possible Side Effects	Considerations Precautions
Opioids	Strong Opioid	Ms Contin	Extended-release. Long-acting with duration of 12 hours.		Can give orally or rectally. Best to use "round-the-clock." *Never crush, break, or cut. * Always awaken patient to give regularly scheduled dose.
	Strong Morphine Derivative	Dilaudid	For moderate to severe pain. Alters perception of and emotional response to pain.	Sedation, dizziness, euphoria, hypotension, nausea, vomiting, constipation, urinary retention, respiratory depression	Comes in tablets, suppositories, syrup, IV, IM, or SQ forms. Pain relief duration approximately four hours.
	Synthetic Opioid	Demerol	Rapid onset and short acting CNS stimulant. Used more for severe acute pain rather than for chronic pain.	Toxicity: mild negative mood swings within 23 hours, irritability, tremors, twitches, seizures	Not drug of choice for terminally ill patient. Is not recommended for chronic pain use due to rapid toxicity.

Commonly Used Medications in a Hospice Setting

Main Category	Sub Category	Example Medications	Uses	Possible Side Effects	Considerations Precautions
Opioids	Non-Morphine Opioid	Fetanyl Transdermal System (Duragesic Patch)	Use for severe pain. For patient who cannot tolerate Morphine. For patients who cannot tolerate anything by mouth.	Sedation, dizziness, euphoria, hypotension, bradycardia, blurred vision, nausea, vomiting, constipation, urine retention	Use with caution for patient with liver or kidney disease. Not for use when frequent titration is required as it may take up to six days to reach equilibrium. Not recommended for fast relief of pain.

Co-Analgesics *given to target specific types of pain*

Type of Pain	Medication Category	Example Medications	Possible Side Effects	Considerations Precautions
Nerve Pain	Trycyclic antidepressant	Elavil Norparamin Pamelor Sinequan Tofranil	Dry mouth, constipation, sedation	Analgesic benefits may take several days to 1-2 weeks. May need to be given at bedtime to reduce daytime sedation effects.
	Anti Convulsant	Tegretol Klonopin Neurontin Dilantin	Dizziness, drowsiness, nausea, headache	If increase in dosage is required, increase gradually. As with Tricyclic antidepressants, pain relief is not immediate.

Co-Analgesics *given to target specific types of pain*

Type of Pain	Medication Category	Example Medications	Possible Side Effects	Considerations Precautions
Nerve Pain	Corticosteroid	Decadron Prednisone	Euphoria, insomnia, seizures, GI irritation, cushingoid effects (moonface, central obesity), CHF, blood clots	Useful in nerve compression pain. Useful in a variety of other symptoms (see chapter). Use cautiously in patients with: stomach or other GI ulcers, kidney or liver disease, high blood pressure, heart disease, seizure disorders, TB, or emotional instability.
Bone Pain		Radiation Therapy	Nausea, vomiting, skin irritation (redness, soreness, burning)	Topical hydrocortisone cream may help with skin soreness. Avoid exposure to sunlight.
	NSAID	Indocin Naprosyn Trilisate Motrin	Dizziness, headache, hypertension, blurred vision, tinnitus, diarrhea, stomach ulcers	Use with caution in patients with kidney or liver disease, heart disease, infection and depression. Give oral dose with food, milk, or antacid to prevent GI problems. First drug of choice for bone pain if radiation therapy cannot be used.
	Corticosteroid	Prednisone Decadron	See above	See above

Co-Analgesics *given to target specific types of pain*

Type of Pain	Medication Category	Example Medications	Possible Side Effects	Considerations Precautions
Gastric Distention Pain	Anti-emetic	Reglan	Restlessness, anxiety, drowsiness, fatigue, confusion	Use cautiously in patients with a history of depression or hypertension.
	Anti-flatulent	Gas-X, Mylanta Phazyme	Simethicone has no major adverse reactions	
Rectal or Bladder Spasm Pain	(Belladona leaf is an anti-cholingeric used to prepare extract and tincture)	B & O suppository (Combination suppository made with Belladona & opium)	Fever due to decreased sweating, vision disturbances, rapid respirations, confusion, dizziness, headache, nausea and vomiting, urine retention, sensitive to light.	Try to keep patient cool due to decreased sweating. Patient may need sunglasses outside if eyes become sensitve to light. If eyes become dry and sensitive use lubricating drops. For dry mouth, use a toothette if patient unable to drink.
	Anti Cholingeric	Cystospaz Levsin	Confusion or excitement in elerly, palpitations, blurred vision, dry mouth, constipation, urinary hesitancy.	Use cautiously in patients with hyperthyroidism, coronary artery disease, congestive heart failure, and high blood pressure. Also use caution with patients in hot or humid environment. Drug-induced heat stroke may develop.
				Use cautiously in patients with liver or kidney impairment

Co-Analgesics *given to target specific types of pain*

Type of Pain	Medication Category	Example Medications	Possible Side Effects	Considerations Precautions
Muscle Spasm Pain	Anti-anxiety	Valium Flexeril	Drowsiness decreased heart rate, decreased respirations	
	Skeletal Muscle Relaxant		Drowsiness, dizziness, dry mouth, seizures	

* Lists are not meant to be all-inclusive. Amount and degree of adverse reactions differ with each individual. Consult a medical professional regarding additional precautions.

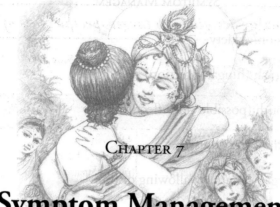

CHAPTER 7

Symptom Management

As a caregiver, you will undoubtedly observe many troublesome symptoms in your patient besides physical pain. This chapter will assist you in recognizing common symptoms experienced by many terminally ill patients, understanding their possible causes, and preparing you to alleviate your patient's discomfort. Depending on the symptoms, intervention may or may not include medications. Often a common sense, back-to-basics approach is sufficient to provide comfort. Even when medications are administered for symptom control, you may wish to use the other suggestions listed under "Back to Basics" to complement the patient's medication regime.

Following is a list of common symptoms often seen in terminally ill patients. Your patient may not show signs of all of these symptoms, but will most likely exhibit some.

Anorexia

Simply stated, anorexia is the lack of interest in food or the lack of desire to eat. Some possible causes include:

- Nausea from medications

- Palliative chemotherapy that sometimes causes a metallic taste in the mouth

- Constipation caused by medications, decreased fluid intake, or immobility

- Depression/anxiety

- Oral thrush (fungal infection)

- Dry mouth (possible side effect from certain types of medications)

- Acid reflux (heartburn)

- Dysphagia (painful swallowing or difficulty when swallowing)

- Early satiety (feeling of fullness) due to hepatomegaly (enlarged liver)

- Declining condition due to disease process

What can be Done?

Medications

Steroids, such as prednisone or dexamethasone (Decadron), are sometimes administered to increase appetite. (Corticosteroids can sometimes increase blood sugar levels and should be used carefully, especially if the patient has a history of diabetes mellitus.) Often an antacid taken one hour before meals is all that is needed if the patient is experiencing heartburn. If oral thrush is the problem, a physician can prescribe an antifungal medication to inhibit fungal growth and enable the patient to swallow more easily. Besides oral thrush, dysphagia can be caused by other factors, such as cancer of the esophagus, radiation therapy to the throat area, or advanced Amyotrophic Lateral Sclerosis. Generally, if a patient is able to swallow saliva without difficulty, he should be able to sip small amounts of liquids. However, alternative routes of medication, other than the oral one, may need to be considered. High-dose steroids can sometimes relieve dysphagia temporarily by reducing inflammation. Laxatives and stool softeners may need to be increased if the patient is experiencing anorexia and/or nausea due to constipation. (The hospice nurse will probably check the patient for fecal impaction.) Senokot and Colace both come in liquid form and may be easier to swallow than tablets. An antidepressant may need to be prescribed if anorexia is caused by severe depression. (Positive effects may not be seen for several weeks.)

Back to Basics

Whether or not the hospice nurse and physician feel it necessary to initiate the use of a medication for your patient's anorexia, the following interventions may be helpful:

- Provide mouth care before meals. This is helpful if the patient has a persistent dry mouth or has altered taste perception due to medications or chemotherapy. Use either a toothbrush or a toothette. Toothettes are foam-stick applicators. Some have a mild mint flavor. Dip the toothette in water and assist the patient in cleansing his mouth.

- Prepare the patient's favorite meals and present them in an attractive manner. A pleasant presentation of a meal can improve appetite.

- Provide meals when the patient desires them, not just at meal times.

- Frequent meals with smaller portions are sometimes more acceptable to patients with anorexia. Simply by seeing large portions on her plate, a patient may experience nausea. If the patient is depressed or is physically weak, attempting to eat large portions may seem like too much of an endeavor.

- Avoid strong-smelling foods, such as cauliflower and cabbage, if the patient is experiencing nausea.

- If a bedside commode is being used, remove it from the room at mealtime.

- Open a window to provide fresh air.

- Avoid strong smells, such as incense and scented candles, during mealtime.

- If the patient has a sore throat or mouth, offer cold foods that are soothing.

- For a dry mouth, provide cool water or another preferred drink at the bedside and freshen it often. Provide a straw if desired and tolerated by the patient.

- Keep a spoon and small ice chips in a cup by the bedside. This is highly recommended when the patient can no longer tolerate drinking liquids. It provides some fluid intake while soothing a dry mouth and throat.

- If the patient is experiencing heartburn, keep him in a sitting position for 30 minutes after eating. Prepare foods that are less spicy. (See antacid information contained in the "Medications" section.)

- If the patient chokes easily while eating, always have her eat in a 90-degree sitting position. Use plenty of pillows, if needed, to prop her up during meals. Be aware of the consistency of foods if choking is a problem. Usually, medium-thick preparations are better tolerated than thin foods, such as soup.

- If the patient is able to walk or be transferred with assistance, eating in a room other than the sickroom may help to increase his appetite.

- Provide smoothies and other liquid supplements that are satisfying as well as nutritious. Below are some suggestions:

High Calorie, High Protein Recipes

High Protein (or Fortified) Milk
1 cup nonfat dry milk powder
1 quart whole milk
Combine ingredients and mix until smooth.

High Protein Shake
½ cup High Protein Milk (see above recipe)
½ cup ice cream
1 tsp vanilla
Place all ingredients in a blender. Blend until smooth.

High Protein Fruit Shake
½ cup High Protein Milk (see above recipe)
¼ cup pureed fruit
Blend until smooth.

Orange Buttermilk Shake
½ cup buttermilk
¼ cup orange juice
1 Tbsp brown sugar
½ cup vanilla ice cream
Blend until smooth.

Peanut Butter Shake
½ cup vanilla ice cream
½ cup half & half
2 Tbsp peanut butter
½ tsp carob powder
Blend until smooth.

Vaishnava Favorites

Hot Milk
1 cup whole milk
2 Tbsp sugar
1 whole cardamom pod
Bring milk to boil. Add sugar and whole cardamom. Simmer for 2-3 minutes. Remove cardamom before serving.

Ginger Tea
2 pints water
3 Tbsp finely grated ginger
4 Tbsp sugar or 3 Tbsp honey
3 Tbsp lemon juice
Boil the water and ginger for about 10-15 minutes. Add sugar and stir. (If using honey, add after tea is strained). Pour though strainer. Add lemon juice. Serve hot.

Lassi

A lassi is a fresh yogurt drink. Often, fresh fruit such as mango is added for a nice flavor and added nutrition. According to *Ayurveda* (India's traditional medical system and part of the *Vedas*), thinning the yogurt by mixing it with water makes it easier to digest.

Sweet Lassi

1 cup fresh yogurt
3-5 cups water
A pinch of ground cardamom
3 Tbsp sugar OR 2 Tbsp honey
A few drops of rosewater (optional)
Mix well in a blender. Add additional sugar or honey to taste.

Fruit Lassi

1 cup fresh berries (strawberries, raspberries, etc.)
⅓ cup sugar
1½ cups plain yogurt
¾ cups water
½ cup crushed ice
Puree berries and sugar and set aside. Place remaining ingredients in blender. Blend until smooth. Add pureed mixture and serve.

Mango-Date Lassi

1 cup fresh yogurt
2-5 cups water
4 chopped dates
1 mango, peeled and pitted
1 pinch ground cardamom
Sugar or honey to taste
Blend until smooth.

High-Nutrient Recipes

Date Milkshake

4-5 whole dates (Medjool variety works well)
1 cup whole milk soymilk, or nut milk

2 pinches of ground cinnamon
Blend until smooth. Serve warm in winter; serve at room temperature or slightly cool, but not cold, in the summer months.

Fresh Cranberry Juice

Cranberries are not only sour, but can be bitter as well. Add sugar or a sweetener of choice to make this juice more flavorful. This fruit has moderate levels of vitamin C, dietary fiber, and other nutrients such as manganese and vitamin K. It is contraindicated for consumption if the patient is taking the medication warfarin, a blood thinner, due to an increased incidence of bruising.

Cranberries contain an antibacterial agent called hippuric acid which acidifies the urine and has long been known for its ability to help treat and prevent urinary tract infections. This tiny fruit reduces the ability of E-coli, the bacteria responsible for 90% of bladder infections, to stick to the bladder wall. Drinking one glass of cranberry juice a day can help reduce the risk of urinary tract infections.

3½ cups fresh cranberries
3½ cups water
1 Tbsp lemon juice
½ cup orange juice or apple juice
⅓ cup sugar or other sweetener of choice to taste

Place cranberries and water in a medium saucepan and bring to a boil. Reduce heat and simmer until the skins on the cranberries open (5 minutes or so). Mash the cranberries slightly and pour through a strainer. Add the remaining ingredients and allow the drink to cool to room temperature before serving.

Green Smoothie
1 Tbsp flax seeds
1 ripe banana
½ can unsweetened pineapple with juice
1 cup tightly packed baby spinach
Water or juice (orange, apple, pineapple) as needed for consistency
Blend until smooth.

Carob Smoothie
1 Tbsp flax seeds
2 ripe bananas
1/4 cup walnuts
5-6 pitted dates
½ tsp vanilla or almond extract
2 Tbsp carob powder
1 cup tightly packed baby spinach
1 cup soymilk, nut milk, or cow's milk
Blend until smooth.

As a caregiver, you may need to explain to loved ones that a patient's appetite will naturally decrease as the disease process worsens. Often, well-meaning family members argue with the patient to eat more because the lack of intake is a harsh reminder that death for the patient is drawing near. Therefore, this struggle is not as much about the patient's decreased appetite as it is about the fear of losing someone dear to them. Eventually, the family will accept the fact that eating and drinking will gradually diminish. In his final days, the terminally ill patient will have no intake at all. He is not starving but simply coming closer to death. This is natural and part of the dying process. During his last days on this earth, Srila Prabhupada exhibited this symptom as well.

Anxiety

A terminally ill patient often experiences some form of anxiety. Anxious feelings may manifest as insomnia, nightmares, rapid breathing and heart rate, tremors, nausea, abdominal pain, headaches, loss of concentration, and irritability. Possible causes of anxiety include:

- Side effects from medications

- Fear of dying

- Actual physical pain or fear of pain

- Anticipatory grieving over present and future losses

- Continued denial (Anxiety can increase if the patient is having a difficult time coping with the harsh reality of his terminal condition. I have seen panic attacks in patients who not only denied their prognosis but denied they were in anxiety, even though many symptoms were present.)

As a patient's condition worsens, the causes of anxiety can be as much physiological as psychological. Possible physical causes include:

- Hypoxia (diminished oxygenation associated with impaired oxygen and CO_2 exchange)

- Dehydration

- Electrolyte imbalance

- Impending cardiac arrest

- Pneumonia

- Arrhythmia (variation in the regular rhythm of the heart)

- Anxious confusion due to disease process, such as brain metastasis

What can be Done?

Medications

For anxious depression, the physician may recommend an antidepressant. Depending on the type of antidepressant medication, benefits may not appear for several weeks. Many patients in hospice care are given an antianxiety medication such as diazepam (Valium), lorazapam (Ativan), or alprazolam (Xanax). Drowsiness is a common side effect with most antianxiety drugs. Oxygen use via nasal cannula may be ordered if the patient's anxiety is due to hypoxia or is causing shortness of breath.

Back to Basics

- Pursed lip breathing: Encourage the patient to *slowly* inhale through his nose and then *slowly* exhale through his mouth while pressing his lips together, leaving a tiny air space. (This exercise works to relax the caregiver as well!) Continue for a few minutes until the patient appears less anxious.

- It may help the patient if you ask, "What are you most worried about?" This often assists her in focusing on the cause of her uneasiness. If she is agreeable, encourage a discussion to help reduce her anxious feelings. Provide reassurance while creating an atmosphere of loving support and acceptance.

- Create a spiritual environment according to the patient's desires. Ultimately, only by being rightly situated in spiritual life can we completely rid ourselves of material anxiety. Offer to play a favorite recording of chanting or bhajans using a low volume. Softly read aloud the scriptures. Chant *japa* together. Become a storyteller. In a calming voice, tell your patient about the Lord's pastimes in Vrindavan. If you, the caregiver, can establish a spiritual, Krishna-conscious atmosphere for your patient, his anxiety will undoubtedly decrease. Hang a favorite picture of Krishna near your patient's bed, or place a photo of his favorite Deities on the bedside table. Encourage him to meditate on rendering devotional service to the Lord.

In the *Nectar of Devotion*, Srila Prabhupada writes, "In the *Visnu-dharma* there is a statement about meditation on the transcendental qualities of the Lord. It is said, 'Persons who are constantly engaged in Krishna consciousness, and who remember the transcendental qualities of the Lord, become free from all reactions to sinful activities, and after being so cleansed they become fit to enter into the kingdom of God.'"

Remind your patient about the story of the *brahmana* and the sweet rice, also in the *Nectar of Devotion*. Srila Prabhupada writes, "In some of the *Puranas* the evidence is given that if someone is simply meditating on devotional activities, he has achieved the desired result and has seen face to face the Supreme Personality of Godhead." A very brief summary of this story from the *Brahma-vaivarta Purana* follows:

> Once there was a poor *brahmana* who lived in the city of Pratishanapura. This humble *brahmana* had nothing materially to offer the Lord. However, after learning that he could meditate on devotional activities and acquire the same results, he lovingly meditated each day on serving the Lord with great opulence. Fixing his consciousness on Krishna, he meditated on dressing the Lord very beautifully with exquisite clothes made of fine cloth. In his mind, he placed opulent jewelry and crowns on the Lord. He then meditated on cleansing the temple, using holy water carried in gold and silver water pots. He continued to meditate on collecting flowers, fruits, incense, and sandalwood pulp to offer to the Deity. The *brahmana* meditated in this way, every day, for many years. One day he meditated on cooking a pot of sweet rice for Lord Krishna. He knew that sweet rice was tastier when eaten cold, so the *brahmana* wanted to touch it to see if it was fit for eating by the Lord. As soon as he meditated on touching the pot, he felt his finger burning in pain. Suddenly, his meditation broke. He opened his eyes and looked at his burnt finger. While this was happening, Lord Vishnu, seated in Vaikuntha, began to smile. The Lord sent a transcendental airplane before the *brahmana* and brought him back home to the spiritual world where he lived eternally in complete knowledge and bliss.

Since devotional service is limited only by our lack of desire to perform it, a terminally ill devotee, although physically incapacitated, can perform the most wonderful service to the Lord without even leaving his bed! This will surely reduce his anxiety.

Bleeding

Minor Bleeding

Minor bleeding includes superficial skin abrasions, skin tears, and lesions. A terminally ill patient with decreased mobility, impaired nutritional status, and whose circulatory system may not be functioning as it once did may exhibit dry, flaky skin that is vulnerable to bruising and abrasions. Minor bleeding from surface areas can usually be controlled by topical measures. Possible causes of minor bleeding may include:

- Disruption of small blood vessels or topical lesions
- Rubbing or other trauma to fragile wound areas
- Incorrect repositioning of the patient resulting in skin tears and abrasions
- Bleeding from the mouth, gums, or nose caused by drying of mucous membranes (can be caused by side effects from medication, chemotherapy, or radiation therapy)

What can be Done?

Medications

Generally, a topical ointment, such as an over-the-counter triple antibiotic ointment, covered with a sterile gauze dressing, is all that is required to prevent infection of superficial skin lesions. ***Every skin irritation, no matter how small, should be brought to the attention of the hospice nurse so it can be assessed and properly treated.*** If nose bleeds due to dryness become a problem, the physician may order a nasal spray to help keep the mucous membranes moist. Nasal dryness and subsequent bleeding can occur if the patient is receiving oxygen via a nasal cannula (nasal prongs). The hospice nurse may recommend humidified oxygen to prevent dryness.

Back to Basics

- If your patient has bleeding, sensitive gums, provide a soft toothbrush or toothette to brush his teeth. Avoid harsh mouthwash that might cause stinging. If he desires to rinse with a mouthwash, dilute a mild mouthwash with lukewarm water.
- For a dry mouth/tongue, mouth care is required every two hours while the patient is awake. It will vary according to the patient's

preference, but mouth care for a hospice patient generally consists of brushing the teeth, rinsing with a diluted mild mouthwash, if appropriate, and applying a lubricant, such as Vaseline ointment, to dry lips to avoid cracking and bleeding. Some patients benefit from rinsing their mouths with a mixture of water and 2% hydrogen peroxide. The taste can be unpleasant, but it is usually effective for cleansing a sore, dry mouth. Dry mouth can be the beginning of oral thrush. Notify the hospice nurse if your patient complains of a dry mouth.

- When giving a bed bath, always use a mild soap and soft cloth. Never rub when drying the skin, but gently pat dry to avoid skin abrasions. Apply a gentle lotion, especially to bony prominences. (See "Skin Care" and "Giving a Bed Bath" in Chapter 8.)

- If you observe a newly developed, minor skin abrasion, cleanse with Normal Saline or with water and a mild soap. Apply an over-the-counter antibiotic ointment and cover with a sterile gauze dressing, using a first-aid paper tape that is gentle on the skin when removed. Cleanse and change the dressing two times a day, or more if it becomes soiled. (I have had patients who were allergic to most types of bandage tape, even the paper type. In these cases, I applied a dab of Vaseline-type ointment on all four corners of the sterile gauze dressing to adhere the dressing to the skin. If you do this, the dressing may need to be replaced more often, but it saves the patient from developing an allergic skin reaction to the tape.) Bring any new skin opening to the attention of the hospice nurse during her next visit.

- Avoid friction rubs against the bottom bed sheet when repositioning or lifting the patient in bed. (See "How to Reposition a Patient" in Chapter 8.)

- Place a cool mist humidifier in the patient's room to add moisture and help reduce drying of nasal passages.

- When a patient is receiving oxygen treatment, never place an oil-based agent, such as Vaseline, in his nostrils in an effort to reduce nasal dryness. It can settle in the lungs and cause pneumonia. As stated above, Vaseline can be applied to dry lips for comfort.

- If your patient has a nosebleed (epistaxis):

1. Remove nasal prongs if the patient is receiving oxygen therapy.

2. Have the patient sit in an upright, 90-degree sitting position with the head slightly bent forward. (Never have the patient bend his head backwards or he can swallow blood.)

3. While he breathes through his mouth, pinch the nostrils just below the bridge of the nose using your thumb and forefinger. Hold for about five minutes. Repeat if the bleeding has not stopped.

4. A cold compress may be applied to the forehead or back of the neck.

5. If the bleeding has not stopped in about 20 minutes, notify the hospice nurse.

- A small amount of bright red rectal bleeding is often a sign of hemorrhoids. Be sure the hospice nurse is made aware of any rectal bleeding, no matter how small an amount. The physician may wish to increase the patient's laxative and stool softener as well as order a suppository to reduce swelling. A warm sitz bath often soothes the burning and discomfort caused by hemorrhoids.

Massive Bleeding

- Some causes of a major bleeding episode may include:

- Cancerous tumor destroying large blood vessels

- Some liver disorders

- Clotting disorders, such as thrombocytopenia (This is a condition caused by the blood containing fewer platelets than normal.

Subsequently, a patient will have a longer bleeding time if she is injured or bleeds for any reason. Thrombocytopenia is a side effect of many drugs, including some chemotherapy medications. Major internal bleeding, or hemorrhaging, can occur if one's platelet count is extremely low.)

Major bleeding episodes may be accompanied by symptoms of anxiety, restlessness, and cool moist skin that appears pale. Notify the hospice nurse if the patient has blood in the urine (hematuria) or bloody stools, is vomiting dark, "coffee-ground" material (hematemesis), has uncontrolled nose bleeds, or any other kind of bleeding. *As a caregiver, always wear latex or other medical gloves when coming in contact with any type of bodily fluid, either directly from the patient or on soiled dressings, clothing, or linens. Properly dispose of waste materials in large, heavy-duty trash bags that are securely tied. Immediately wash your hands with a disinfectant soap and water after handling soiled material.*

It may be upsetting to the patient and family members to see large amounts of blood. If there is even the slightest possibility that your patient may have a major bleeding episode, have on hand an "Emergency Kit" containing some red or dark colored towels to cover the blood, some dark washcloths, a small wash basin, a large plastic bag to put the used towels in, and a plastic cover to protect the bed. (I have used a new shower curtain liner. They are inexpensive and large enough to cover a twin or full size mattress.) Call the hospice nurse. **DO NOT CALL 911 OR YOUR LOCAL EMERGENCY MEDICAL HOTLINE.** Stay calm and relax the patient while waiting for the nurse to arrive.

Constipation

Constipation means difficult, irregular stools and is experienced by the majority of terminally ill patients. Prevention, by treating it as a problem before it becomes one, is a challenge all caregivers must confront. Patients will complain of hard-formed stools, inability to pass stool for at least two to three days, seepage of a small amount of liquid stool (diarrhea leaking past the fecal mass), and mild to moderately tender abdominal distention. Constipation is often accompanied by nausea and vomiting. It can also cause anorexia, rectal pain, and confusion. Each individual varies but, as a general rule, a patient should have a bowel movement at least every three days. Constipation can lead to painful hemorrhoids as well as to fecal impaction (stool that remains in the rectum and is unable to be evacuated). The nurse usually has to disimpact the patient by manually emptying the rectum. This can be extremely uncomfortable for the patient, sometimes requiring administration of a pain medication before the procedure is performed. Occasionally, the impaction is higher up and hospitalization may be necessary to clear this type of complication. Even more serious is a bowel obstruction (stool that collects higher in the intestines). Therefore, it is recommended that the caregiver keep a written record of the patient's bowel movements. This may seem unpleasant, but the medical consequences of prolonged constipation are even more unpleasant. Common causes of constipation include:

- Side effects of medications, especially opioids, anti-cholinergics, and tricyclic antidepressants

- Decreased mobility

- Decreased fluid intake that reduces fluid in the colon

- Decreased fiber intake

- Dehydration

- Improper use of laxatives, especially when taking opioids (either intermittent use or inadequate amount of laxatives)

What can be done?

Medications

As soon as any type of opioid is started, a laxative and stool softener regimen must be started immediately. If the laxative dose is too low or it is administered only intermittently, the patient will still experience constipation. Every hospice differs in its protocol and choice of bowel medications. There are, however, bowel medications that are more commonly used than others. Two effective medications that combine a laxative and a stool softener are

Senokot-S (senna and docusate sodium) and Peri-Colace (docusate sodium and casanthranol). Senokot (senna) is a laxative only without the stool softener and Colace (docusate sodium) is a stool softener only without the laxative. Taking it in combination form is obviously more convenient and decreases the amount of pills that need to be swallowed by the patient. Milk of Magnesia is usually administered at bedtime with a large glass of water, either as needed when already taking a regularly-scheduled laxative or routinely as part of the medication schedule. Bisacodyl suppositories (e.g., Dulcolax) are commonly used in a hospice setting. One or two suppositories are usually effective within an hour. Castor oil taken orally (it now comes flavored) is also an effective stool softener. A bulk-forming agent, such as psyllium (e.g., Metamucil) should only be taken if the patient is drinking an adequate amount of fluid. Otherwise, it tends to increase the incidence of fecal impaction. If the patient becomes impacted, the hospice nurse may administer a Mineral Oil Retention Enema prior to disimpacting the patient. He or she may follow up with a Fleets Enema or a normal saline enema. Some nurses prefer to administer a milk and molasses enema. (The formula is four cups of warm water mixed with one cup of powdered milk and one cup of molasses.)

Back to Basics

Encourage an increase in fluids. Keep a pitcher of fresh water at the bedside.

- Serve warm prune juice.

- Encourage intake of fiber-filled foods, such as bran. (Bran should only be taken if the patient is drinking a lot of fluids. Otherwise, it will be counter-productive.)

- Encourage an increase in fruits and vegetables. If the patient is experiencing anorexia, serve various fruit and vegetable juices. Make "ice pops" by pouring fruit juice in paper cups. Place a spoon in each cup and freeze.

- If possible, encourage the patient to walk, even if he just walks around the room once or twice. (If he is bedridden, simply by repositioning the patient every two hours, he will receive some benefits of mobilization.)

- Serve high-fiber breads and cereals, such as oatmeal.

Diarrhea

Diarrhea, frequent loose or liquid bowel movements, is less common in hospice patients than constipation. It does occur, though, and can be accompanied by painful abdominal cramping. Causes may include:

- Incorrect dose of laxatives and stool softeners
- Undetected fecal impaction
- Early bowel obstruction
- Side effects of chemotherapy
- Side effects of medications, such as antibiotics and some NSAIDs
- An intestinal obstruction caused by malignancy
- Steatorrhea (pale, floating, loose stools caused by the malabsorption of fat, commonly seen in patients with pancreatic cancer)
- Diet, including lactose intolerance
- Pre-existing conditions, such as colitis or irritable bowel syndrome, that may exacerbate with anxiety and fear

What can be Done?

Medications

A patient should never be medicated for diarrhea if a bowel obstruction is suspected. If the patient has steatorrhea, the condition may respond to pancreatic enzyme replacement therapy (lipase, protease, and amylase). Loperamide (e.g., Imodium) is often given for diarrhea even when the cause may be a malignant intestinal obstruction. (The steroid dexamethasone can also be administered for this situation.) Pepto-Bismol and Kaopectate are often administered to hospice patients as well. If Imodium, Pepto-Bismol, and Kaopectate are ineffective, a prescription for diphenoxylate (Lomotil) is sometimes obtained. It is essential to balance a patient's laxative use so she does not get caught in the cycle of constipation (caused by under medication with laxatives) and diarrhea (caused by over medication with laxatives). Use of laxatives and stool softeners can be tricky and may require frequent adjustments.

Back to Basics

- Stop administering laxatives and other bowel medications until the diarrhea has stopped. (Inquire from the hospice nurse about other medications being taken that may cause diarrhea as a side effect.)

- Stop food supplements, such as milk shakes, that may cause diarrhea.

- Serve a "clear liquid diet" only until the diarrhea has stopped. Serve clear juices, such as apple juice; soda, such as ginger ale; clear vegetable broth; water; or an electrolyte-balancing sports drink. (As a rule of thumb, a "clear liquid diet" is anything that you can clearly see through.)

- Avoid milk products, non-clear soups, and non-clear juices. Never give prune juice when the patient is experiencing diarrhea.

- When diarrhea ceases, slowly increase diet to full liquids, such as cream soup. Increase diet as tolerated to a soft diet and then to a regular diet. The patient's hospice nurse or physician should advise you as to when to restart the patient's bowel medications.

- If certain foods, such as products containing lactose, are causing diarrhea, keeping a food diary should help to solve the mystery. Keep a daily log of all foods that are eaten by the patient and when. Also, list each time the patient had diarrhea after eating. A pattern should begin to appear as to what foods, if any, cause diarrhea.

- Immaculate skin care is especially important when a patient has diarrhea because he is at high risk for developing soreness, redness, or rash on the buttocks. If he is able to shower or bathe without assistance, provide a mild soap and encourage him to pat dry the area of concern, rather than rub dry, to decrease his chances of soreness. Whether the patient is independent with bathing or requires assistance, after drying, the caregiver should apply a thick cream to the buttock area to protect the skin. (When in the U.S. I prefer Balmex Cream. It helps shield the skin from moisture, is inexpensive, stays on for several hours, and a little goes a long way. It can be found at most grocery or drug stores.)

Dyspnea

Dyspnea means labored or difficult breathing. This may or may not be accompanied by pain but is always distressing to the patient and to those watching. The patient may exhibit shortness of breath on exertion or at rest. Dyspnea may be accompanied by cyanosis, a bluish discoloration of the skin and/or lips. Onset of dyspnea may be sudden or gradual and may or may not be accompanied by a cough. Causes may include:

- Extreme fatigue

- Pulmonary (lung) disease interfering with air exchange, such as Chronic Obstructive Pulmonary Disease (COPD) or lung cancer (either as the primary site of cancer or as lung metastasis). A growing tumor will usually cause gradual onset of dyspnea.

- Infection, such as pneumonia

- Pulmonary embolus (An obstruction in the pulmonary artery, usually caused by a blood clot that has broken away from a lower extremity. This causes sudden onset of dyspnea. I have seen a few patients die suddenly when this occurred. Although it is an extremely serious condition, it is not always fatal.)

- Heart failure resulting in pulmonary edema (This causes sudden onset of dyspnea.)

- Anxiety (may cause sudden hyperventilation)

- Anemia (Low number of circulating red blood cells. Hemoglobin, the iron-containing component of the red blood cell, is less than that needed to supply the body's oxygen demands. Anemia usually causes gradual onset of dyspnea. The patient may become cyanotic.)

What can be Done?

Medications

In a hospice setting, fast-acting liquid morphine sulfate is usually the drug of choice for severe shortness of breath. Often, a low dose of instant/immediate release morphine is all that is needed to decrease respirations and assist in making each breath more efficient. For dyspnea, morphine can also be administered via a nebulizer, a small device that produces a fine mist which is then inhaled. The nebulization of opioids delivers medication directly into the airways, thus entering the pulmonary circulation quickly. Advocates state that this route of administration causes fewer adverse effects, such as drowsiness, nausea, vomiting, and constipation.

An antianxiety medication, such as lorazapam (e.g., Ativan), can be dissolved under the tongue if dyspnea is caused by sudden feelings of panic. Lorazapam is also available in gel form, to be applied directly to the skin. Some patients respond well to diazepam (e.g., Valium). Bronchodilators, such as ipratropium bromide (Atrovent) or albuterol (e.g., Ventolin), are often helpful and can be administered through an inhaler. Theophylline (e.g., Theo-Dur), also a bronchodilator, is commonly used when dyspnea is caused by COPD. If dyspnea is caused by cardiac failure, the physician may prescribe a diuretic. Antibiotics may be needed if the patient has an infection, such as bacterial pneumonia. (If the patient is responsive, be sure to ask him if he agrees to the use of antibiotics in the case of infection and if used for comfort. If he is unresponsive, abide by his wishes as stated in his living will.)

Back to Basics

- If the patient is in a hospital bed, the head of the bed should be raised to a 45-90 degree angle so the patient is in a sitting position. If she is not using a hospital bed, assist the patient in a sitting position by propping enough pillows behind her so her head and chest are raised.

- Reassure the patient that you will not leave her alone.

- If the patient is using oxygen therapy, be sure the nasal prongs are inserted properly. In a calm voice, remind her to "feel" the oxygen being inhaled with each breath.

- Provide a gentle breeze toward the patient's face by opening a window, using a small electric fan (turned on low and facing the patient), or using a cool mist vaporizer (if dyspnea is accompanied by cough).

- While the patient is in a sitting position, assist him in pursed lip breathing (see "Anxiety"). Try to relax the patient with your calming voice as you talk him through this breathing technique. As he slows his respirations, perform pursed lip breathing with him. Then, try slowly chanting the *maha-mantra* as he continues to use this breathing technique, or assist the patient in a meditation that will relax his mind and assist in slowing respirations.

Edema

Edema is swelling due to body tissues containing an excessive amount of fluid. It can be local or generalized. A patient may exhibit peripheral edema of the extremities, most often in the feet and ankles. Pitting edema refers to an indentation maintained in the swollen area after being pressed with the finger. It is measured by the numbers 1-4, corresponding to the depth of the depression left in the skin. Number 1+ means the indentation is barely noticeable, 2+ means the indentation is less than 5 mm, 3+ means the indentation is 5-10 mm, and 4+ means the indentation is greater than 10 mm in depth. In severe cases of edema, the skin will appear taut and shiny with weeping of clear fluid usually seen in small droplets on the skin. It is not unusual for a terminally ill patient to exhibit some type of edema as the systems of the body begin to shut down.

Lymphedema in the upper or lower extremities is exhibited by painful swelling. The skin sometimes appears slightly red and may be extremely painful to the patient when touched. Lymphedema in the arms and hands is often associated with breast cancer that has metastasized to the lymph nodes or with radiation therapy to the axilla (underarm) area. It can also occur after a mastectomy. Lymphedema is caused by an accumulation of protein-filled fluid in the limb due to damaged or blocked lymph nodes that are unable to perform their task of carrying this fluid throughout the lymphatic system. The limb that is edematous is highly susceptible to infection and care must be taken to avoid cuts, shearing, or burns.

When caring for my mother-in-law with metastatic breast cancer, she exhibited severe lymphedema in her right arm due to radiation therapy and metastasis to the axillary lymph nodes. She also exhibited lymphedema in her legs due to a tumor in the pelvis. Her right arm edema was controlled for a few months by regular lymphedema massage by a trained physical therapist and by a lengthy process of daily wrapping her fingers and arms with layers of soft cotton gauze, a compression stocking, and foam. In her final days, however, this process became more painful than the lymphedema itself. At this point, I simply elevated her arm on a soft pillow for comfort.

Other causes of edema (excluding lymphedema) may include:

- Hypoproteinemia (a decrease in the amount of protein in the blood)

- Excessive salt intake

- Fluid-retaining medications (steroids, NSAIDS, or tamoxifen citrate, sometimes administered for breast cancer)

- Decreased cardiac output

- Impaired kidney function

- Fluid overload from intravenous or tube feedings (see "Dehydration" section below)

- Phlebitis (inflammation of a vein, causing localized pain, warmth at the site, and swelling)

- Cellulitis (inflammation of cellular or connective tissue that spreads through the tissue, causing redness, swelling, and, if severe, weeping of fluid through the skin)

What can be Done?

Medications

The physician may consider changing a medication that causes fluid retention. Diuretics are sometimes recommended, depending on the cause of the edema. A potassium supplement may be added to the patient's medication regime, depending on the type of diuretic prescribed. Diuretics will naturally cause the patient to urinate more often, sometimes creating a problem of inconvenience, especially when it disturbs sleep. If incontinence is a consideration, the caregiver will need to pay special attention to skin care, cleansing the patient often and keeping the skin dry. An indwelling urinary catheter may need to be considered when diuretics are used. A catheter helps to keep the skin dry and free from rashes and other irritations caused by urinary incontinence. It also allows the patient to rest without the inconvenience of frequent urination. (The main risk of having a urinary catheter inserted is developing a urinary tract infection.) Diuretics are not recommended for lymphedema. Antibiotics are sometimes recommended if cellulitis is present.

Back to Basics

- Unless otherwise instructed by the physician, place pillows comfortably under edematous legs and feet or if a hospital bed is being used, raise the lower portion so extremities are elevated. Either way, the legs should be raised to the level of the heart in order to be effective in reducing edema. Reposition the pillows and the patient's extremities every two hours as tolerated or sooner if the patient desires.

- If edema is in the hand or arm (as in lymphedema), gently place a pillow under the edematous limb for comfort and to help reduce swelling.

- Turn and reposition the patient every two hours as tolerated or sooner if the patient desires. Consult with the hospice nurse on proper repositioning when lymphedema is present.

- Decrease added salt when preparing meals.

- Encourage natural diuretics, such as hot herbal tea, if tolerated.

- If taking diuretics, encourage potassium-rich foods, such as bananas and orange juice. (However, first discuss this with the physician or hospice nurse to see if it is advisable. Increased potassium may be contraindicated in certain conditions, such as kidney failure.)

- Advise the patient to avoid sitting upright for long periods with legs dangling. This will increase dependent edema in lower extremities.

- Ask the physician or hospice nurse if compression stockings are indicated.

Fever

A fever is an elevation of body temperature above the normal temperature. In general, a person's temperature is considered within normal range if it is one degree above or one to two degrees below the normal temperature. Body temperature is usually lower in the morning and higher in the late afternoon/evening. Symptoms of fever may include flushed hot skin (skin may initially feel cool at onset of fever), headache, generalized aching in the muscles and/or joints (may suggest a viral infection), increased respirations and heartbeat, increased thirst, decreased urine output, weakness, and chills. Coughing which produces rust-colored or yellowish phlegm and/or wheezing may suggest pneumonia or other pulmonary infection. Vomiting and/or diarrhea when a fever is present may suggest an infection of the digestive tract.

Normal oral temperatures are as listed below:

	Celsius	Fahrenheit
Infant	36-38 degrees	97-100 degrees
Child	37 degrees	98.6 degrees
Adult	37 degrees	98.6 degrees
Elderly	36 degrees	98 degrees

To convert Celsius to Fahrenheit: F = (Celsius x 9/5) + 32
To convert Fahrenheit to Celsius: C = (Fahrenheit minus 32) x 5/9

In a patient who is terminally ill, possible causes of fever include:

- Infection, such as an infected wound or urinary tract infection

- Pneumonia

- "Tumor fever" (Tumor fevers are often seen with liver metastasis. Also, tumors in the central nervous system, such as a brain tumor, often cause a persistent fever that is either elevated or remains low-grade.)

- Toxic effects of some medications

- End-stage disease process

A patient's temperature can be taken orally, axillary (under arm), rectally, or by a tympanic (ear) thermometer. The oral temperature is the patient's accurate body temperature. However, if the patient is unconscious or is unable to tolerate having a thermometer in her mouth, temperature should be taken either under the arm, rectally, or with a tympanic thermometer. From my experience, temperature strip thermometers can be costly and their accuracy can fluctuate.

Mercury thermometers are no longer manufactured in the U.S.; however, if you are using one, carefully shake the thermometer so the mercury falls below the normal mark (98.6 degrees Fahrenheit/37 degrees Celsius). Wash it with cool water. Place it under the tongue and leave the thermometer in place for 3-5 minutes with the patient's mouth closed.

For better accuracy, it is best to wait at least 15-20 minutes after the patient has eaten or has had a hot or cold drink before taking an oral temperature. The same applies if the patient has just had a bath or shower.

When taking an axillary temperature, place the tip of the thermometer in the armpit of the patient. Then lower the patient's arm close to his side to hold the thermometer in place for approximately 8-10 minutes. *Add* one degree Fahrenheit (0.5 degrees Celsius) to convert to the oral temperature.

When taking a temperature rectally, insert the thermometer only 1½ inches with an adult patient and only 1 inch with a child. Hold in place for two to four minutes. *Subtract* one degree Fahrenheit (0.5 degrees Celsius) to convert to the oral temperature.

Digital thermometers are used in the same way as the "old-fashioned" glass thermometers but register in much less time (usually about one minute.)

Tympanic thermometers are held against the inside of the ear and usually register in about 2-3 seconds.

What can be Done?

Medications

Acetaminophen (e.g., Tylenol or Paracetamol) is usually recommended to reduce a fever. If the patient is unable to swallow tablets, the physician can prescribe acetaminophen suppositories to be administered rectally. If it is determined that the patient has an infection, such as a urinary tract infection, the physician will probably prescribe an antibiotic. If the patient has an infected wound, a combination of systemic antibiotics, as well as wound care with a topical antibiotic, may be prescribed.

Back to Basics

Once it is established that the fever is not caused by an infection, or if the source of infection has been determined and appropriate medications have been prescribed, the following measures can be taken to help reduce the fever:

- Encourage the patient to wear lightweight, loose-fitting clothing.

- Unless requested by the patient, do not bundle him under heavy blankets in an attempt to "sweat out the fever." Remove blankets and loosely cover the patient with a cotton sheet. Rather than tucking in the sheet, it can be "tented" by placing the edges over the side rails of a hospital bed. If a hospital bed is not being used, place pillows and drape the sheet over the patient with the edges of the sheet "tented" over the pillows.

- Provide circulating room air. Do not direct a fan or air conditioner directly toward the patient.

- Provide sponge baths with lukewarm water. (See "Giving a Bed Bath" in Chapter 8.) Never use rubbing alcohol on the patient to reduce a fever, because it tends to cool the patient's body temperature too quickly. It also has a very strong odor and has a drying effect on the skin.

- Place a cool, moist washcloth on the patient's forehead. For a fever over 102 degrees Fahrenheit or 38.8 Celsius, place small ice packs in the axilla under both arms and in the groin area to reduce fever. Be sure to cover the ice packs in cotton cloth before placing against the skin.

- If tolerated, encourage an increase in fluids, such as water, juices, ice chips, or fruit pops.

- As the patient's temperature decreases, he will probably perspire a great deal. Assist in keeping the skin clean and dry. As bed sheets become moist, change them as needed for the patient's comfort.

- The patient's mouth may tend to become dry with a fever. Using a moist toothette, perform mouth care every two hours or more as needed.

Nausea and Vomiting

With a terminal illness, nausea can occur without vomiting, and vomiting may occur spontaneously without warning of nausea. Briefly, there is a part of the midbrain where the vomiting center is located. Here the brain receives messages from the cerebral cortex (signals anxiety), the inner ear (signals vertigo), the chemoreceptor trigger zone (signals toxins in the blood, such as chemotherapy and other drugs), and the gastrointestinal tract (signals peptic ulcer or other stomach/intestinal upset). Causes of nausea and/or vomiting vary and may include:

- Anxiety

- Medication reaction, especially with opioids, NSAIDs, antibiotics, estrogens, and chemotherapy

- Primary brain tumor or brain metastasis

- Constipation and/or fecal impaction

- Bowel obstruction

- Motion sickness (can occur with inner ear infections)

- Stomach ulcer or gastrointestinal infection

- Abdominal carcinoma

- Excessive coughing with mucous production

What can be Done?

Medications

As a caregiver, keep an accurate record of when your patient experiences nausea and/or vomiting. This will aid the physician and hospice nurse in evaluating the cause. Does the patient have nausea without vomiting? Does the patient have strong projectile vomiting without warning of nausea? Is the emesis bright red? Is it coffee-ground-looking material? (The latter may indicate a gastrointestinal bleed.) Is there a pattern of any sensory stimulation that causes nausea, such as cooking smells, incense, etc.? Are the caregivers turning the patient too quickly, causing dizziness and nausea? Does the patient consistently vomit after taking an opioid for pain? In that case, the physician may adjust the dose or prescribe an alternate pain medication. Similarly, some NSAIDs can cause nausea and vomiting. If this occurs, switching to another NSAID on a trial basis may be helpful because the patient may not react the same to all NSAIDs. Antibiotics given for symptom management, as in the case of a urinary tract infection, can sometimes cause nausea and vomiting. Again, a patient may have this side effect with one antibiotic and not another. If the cause of nausea or vomiting is constipation, a change or an increase in the patient's daily laxative regime may be helpful. If anxiety is so great that it is causing nausea and/or vomiting, the patient may benefit from an antianxiety medication when anxiousness is at its worst. If a patient's nausea is caused by raised intracranial pressure, as is sometimes the case with a brain tumor, he may benefit from a steroid, such as dexamethasone, to decrease inflammation.

Usually the physician will prescribe an antiemetic, depending on the cause of the patient's nausea or vomiting. As previously stated, when a patient begins an opioid for pain management, an antiemetic should always be prescribed on an as-needed basis for nausea and/or vomiting. A patient may be especially vulnerable to these side effects during the first few days of taking morphine. In this case, an antiemetic is sometimes prescribed round the clock during the first few days while the patient adjusts to the strong opioid. If for any reason nausea persists and becomes severe, then two or more different kinds of antiemetics may be required because each drug will act to subdue nausea at a different site. For example, Haloperidol

(Haldol) is recommended as an antiemetic when the chemoreceptor signal zone triggers nausea due to toxins in the body. Procholorperazine (Compazine) is recommended for nausea with or without vomiting being present. It also acts on the chemoreceptor signal zone. Procholorperazine, as well as other antiemetics, are available in suppository form to be given rectally when the patient can no longer swallow medication or is unable to keep it down due to nausea and vomiting.

Back to Basics

Aside from using the appropriate medications, these suggestions may help provide comfort for your patient:

- Give antiemetics 30 minutes before meals or as prescribed by the physician.

- Provide good oral hygiene for the patient before and after meals so the mouth feels clean. The often helps to alleviate nausea.

- Avoid movements that produce nausea.

- Do not serve foods with harsh smells, such as cabbage, that may exacerbate nausea. (When someone is nauseous, even subtle odors can cause one to become ill.) Prepare bland foods and clear liquids until the nausea subsides.

- Offer small meals rather than large, hearty meals.

- If the patient is vomiting with nausea, ask the hospice nurse or physician for diet instructions.

- Keep a cup of small chipped ice by the bedside with a teaspoon. If the patient is weak, offer to feed her only one or two small ice chips at a time. This will help avoid dehydration.

- Sometimes small sips of clear carbonated soda or carbonated water can be tolerated with nausea. This will also help avoid dehydration.

- Be aware that fragrant candles, incense, or fresh flowers can cause the patient to experience nausea.

- Provide dim lighting when the patient is feeling nausea and/or vomiting.

- Provide a relaxed environment by decreasing environmental stimuli.

- Encourage the patient to rest after meals.

- Provide good oral hygiene for the patient throughout the day, especially if the patient is experiencing a dry mouth with thick secretions.

- Remove any unsightly items in the room, such as a bedside commode, to create a more pleasant atmosphere during meals.

- If your patient begins to vomit while lying on his back, immediately roll him over to a side-lying position so the contents are not aspirated into the lungs. If possible, assist him to a sitting position with head bent slightly forward.

Dehydration versus Intravenous Fluid

I have seen countless families suffer great anguish when a loved one slowly stops eating and drinking until, finally, there is no intake at all. The issue of whether or not to offer IV hydration to a terminally ill patient who is nearing death is a sensitive, and often controversial, one. Many family members feel tremendous guilt and turmoil when deciding to withhold artificial hydration.

"He is starving to death," many have said, with panic in their voices. "I can't get him to take even one bite."

These emotions are natural. It is heart wrenching to watch someone we care about physically waste away before our eyes. We are sure they are suffering from hunger and thirst. It is also a constant reminder that death for the patient is near. In some hospitals it is standard protocol to provide hydration through intravenous (IV) fluids, even when the patient is near death. I have even seen physicians convince relatives that a gastric tube surgically inserted into the dying patient's stomach would be best so liquid supplements could then be administered. In this section, I will examine both sides of the controversy surrounding dehydration versus IV fluids for the terminally ill in order for the patient, caregiver, and other loved ones to determine what is best for your particular situation.

Physiology of the Terminally Ill Patient

"Terminal dehydration" occurs when a dying patient naturally loses interest in and ability to eat and drink. Within days before imminent death, a lack of fluid intake causes reduced circulation in all body systems. Your patient may experience internal bleeding, drainage from wounds, diarrhea, and vomiting, all of which can contribute to fluid loss as well as an electrolyte imbalance. A patient with an electrolyte imbalance can exhibit twitching and restlessness due to neuromuscular irritability. Confusion and disorientation often follow. A decrease in consciousness, with or without terminal dehydration, is often inevitable at the end stage of a terminal illness.

However, it is important to remember that the physiology of a strong, healthy individual who is deprived of food and drink is entirely different from that of a dying person. As difficult as it is to watch, your patient's desire and need for sustenance will decrease as a natural part of the disease process. Emotional withdrawal from this world may play a key part, as well.

Benefits of Dehydration

Dehydration in a terminally ill patient who is close to death can actually relieve some distressing symptoms. In addition, some studies conclude that blood chemistry alteration resulting from terminal dehydration produces a natural anesthesia for the central nervous system in the final days of life. (This does not mean that pain medications should be stopped.) However, the exact mechanism of this process is still unclear. Other significant benefits are as follows:

- Decreased urine output can decrease the need for an indwelling urinary catheter, bedpans, bedside commode, or adult diaper changes if the patient is incontinent. Especially if incontinence is a problem, this will decrease the chances of skin breakdown, such as a rash.

- Decreased gastrointestinal fluid will diminish bouts of nausea and vomiting, especially if the patient has a bowel obstruction.

- Decreased pulmonary secretions can reduce associated cough and congestion.

- Decrease in pharyngeal secretions (at the back of the throat) can bring relief to the patient who has had difficulty swallowing secretions, even to the point of choking on his own saliva. A decrease in these secretions may diminish the patient's "drowning" sensation.

- Decrease in body fluid will cause peripheral (limb) edema to lessen. Arms and legs will appear less swollen, bringing relief to the tightness and discomfort edema can cause. A patient who has had edema surrounding a tumor, in the abdomen for example, may experience a reabsorption of the fluid in the last days with reduction and relief from pressure sensation.

Difficulties Caused by Dehydration

Dry mouth seems to be the most significant hardship caused by dehydration in the terminally ill patient. (Remember that medications can also contribute to dry mouth.) Thickened secretions often coat the inside of the mouth.

What Can Be Done?

The following interventions can provide relief for your patient:

- Provide excellent mouth care every two hours or more often as needed. Keep a pitcher of fresh water by the bedside. Pour into a cup and dip a fresh sponge toothette (or very soft toothbrush) into the water. Squeeze any excess water off the toothette or toothbrush.

Even a few drops of water may cause the patient to choke. Gently swab the patient's tongue, gums, teeth, and lips. Be sure to wipe the upper palate with the toothette. Secretions and other debris can accumulate in this area of the mouth.

- A few drops of a mild, fresh-tasting, alcohol-free mouthwash may be added to the water before cleansing the mouth.

- If the patient can tolerate the taste, dilute water with hydrogen peroxide to thoroughly cleanse the mouth from debris.

- Do not use premoistened lemon and glycerin swabs for mouth care, as these cause excessive dryness.

- If the patient is still conscious and able to swallow small amounts, use a teaspoon to offer one small ice chip at a time. If the patient is too weak to sip through a straw, or the use of a straw causes him to choke, spoon-feed a few drops of liquid at a time. Go slowly. Swallowing will be an endeavor at this point. I sometimes place a straw in a cup of water, holding my finger over the top of the straw. I then place the straw in the patient's mouth, lifting my finger up and down from the top opening of the straw. In this way I can control the amount of liquid being swallowed by my patient.

- Moisten lips with lip balm or another protective coating to avoid dryness and cracking.

Neuromuscular irritability and twitching, as mentioned above, confusion, and nausea are other concerns with dehydration. Sedatives and antiemetics may help to alleviate these problems, should they arise.

Benefits of Intravenous Fluid

It is uncommon for a hospice patient to be given IV fluids close to death. However, if the family and physician decide to initiate artificial hydration, IV fluids can correct electrolyte imbalances. This may result in a temporary increase in consciousness, a decrease in restlessness, a decrease in nausea, and stabilization of cardiac arrhythmias, if these have been a problem.

This improvement in your patient's condition may appear to prolong life, but because of his disease condition, death is unavoidable. It is essential to consider the patient's wishes, either previously verbalized or written in his living will. It is also important to measure the quality of life that is being prolonged by the use of artificial hydration.

Detrimental Effects of Intravenous Fluid

Initiating artificial hydration at the end of one's life can result in discomfort for the patient and emotional distress for the family. I once cared for an elderly lady who was unconscious and nearing death. Her adult daughter, out of love, could not bear the thought of her mother "starving to death." She insisted on IV fluids round the clock, thinking this would comfort her mother. One day, while visiting in the hospice inpatient unit, she noticed that her mother's arms and legs were extremely swollen. Every breath was an effort, and she sounded as if she were drowning. Crying, the daughter expressed regret for her decision to artificially hydrate her mother with IV fluids. "Please pull the IV out," she begged. "I now understand what you were trying to tell me." Her mother never regained consciousness, in spite of being given IV fluids. Days later, she died more comfortably, without IV fluids being administered.

The following effects may occur when artificial hydration is administered during the end-stage disease process:

- Increased urination, possibly requiring the insertion of an indwelling urinary catheter with increased risk of infection

- Increased gastrointestinal tract fluid possibly causing vomiting, especially if the patient has a bowel obstruction

- Increased pulmonary secretions causing moist respirations, choking, and coughing

- Edema (swelling in the limbs)

- An increase in wound drainage

- Excess fluid can expand the edematous layer around a tumor and place pressure on surrounding organs.

In conclusion, it is never easy for caregivers and family members to confront the issue of dehydration of a loved one. It is frustrating to watch, and feelings of helplessness are common. Every patient is different, and each situation requires thoughtful consideration. Hopefully, the patient will have made this decision while he was still able to verbalize his wishes. If not, though he may be silent now, he can still voice his desires through his advance directives as written in his living will. As a caregiver, reassure the family that they are not the ones making the decision. Whatever the patient previously decided should now be heard and honored.

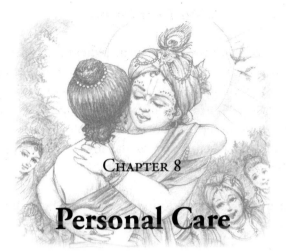

Chapter 8

Personal Care

The following offers practical suggestions on caring for the personal needs of a terminally ill patient. These are general guidelines. Naturally, ways of providing care will vary and adjustments will need to be made according to the individual needs of your patient, his or her wishes, and the physical environment in which you are working.

Giving a Bed Bath

A comforting bed bath can lift the spirits and provide an overall feeling of well-being. A patient who is bedridden becomes stiff and sore from immobility and the skin often feels moist. A warm bath can refresh the skin and soothe tired muscles and joints. One of my favorite rewards of being a caregiver is watching the transformation on my patient's face after she has been cleansed and revitalized.

1) Fill a washbasin with warm water and a small amount of a mild, liquid soap. Have two or three washcloths available, as well as three large towels (one will be used under the patient, one will be used to cover the patient, and one will be used to dry the patient.) Have latex or other medical gloves available.

2) Be sure the room is warm before undressing the patient and starting a bath. Close all windows if a draft will cause a chill. Turn off fans or air conditioner.

3) Place a large bath towel under the patient to protect the sheet and mattress. If the patient is unable to turn by himself, assist by "log-rolling" him, meaning the entire body is rolled to a side-lying position with one smooth motion. Roll the towel lengthwise and tuck about half of the towel under the patient. "Log-roll" the patient to his other side and unroll the remainder of the towel. Roll the patient on his back so the towel is centered under him.

4) Remove the patient's clothing and cover her with a large bath towel (a folded sheet will work just as well).

5) After putting on gloves, wash the patient's face, ears, and neck (and scalp if you are not going to wash his hair). Gently dry with the towel. Wash his chest, abdomen, arms, and underarms, rinsing the washcloth often in the basin. Gently pat the skin dry. Uncover only the part of the body you are washing to maintain your patient's dignity and to prevent a chill. Wash and dry his legs and feet in the same manner.

6) Roll your patient to a side-lying position to wash and dry her back.

7) If the patient is conscious, it is very comforting for him to dip his hands in a basin of warm water for a minute or two. Dry them with a towel.

8) Again, if the patient is conscious, assist her in bending her knees so her feet are flat on the bed. Gently lift each foot and place it in the basin of warm water, one at a time. Have a towel placed at the foot of the bed to protect the sheet. Leave each foot in the water for a minute or two. Dry each foot carefully, especially between the toes. This is most refreshing for a bedridden patient and provides relaxation as well.

9) If the patient is able, provide him with a moist washcloth and dry towel and ask him to cleanse his private areas, front and back. Provide a few minutes of privacy to maintain your patient's dignity. If he is unable, a caregiver must provide excellent care for him, in order

to avoid infections and skin rashes. Always pat dry, especially if the patient has a rash or any openings in the skin. If applicable, apply lotion (or any prescribed ointments) to the buttocks as a moisture barrier.

10) Finally, after washing your hands, apply a moisturizing lotion to the patient's face, neck, arms, legs, and feet, if applicable. Assist your patient with dressing in clean clothes or nightclothes.

11) As a final touch after giving a bed bath, comb or brush your patient's hair, reposition her for comfort using fresh, clean pillows, and cover her with a clean top sheet and blanket.

Washing your Patient's Hair

Even if your patient is bedridden, it is still possible to wash his or her hair. The following suggestions should help:

1) Place a large piece of plastic (I use a large trash bag) under the patient to protect the bottom bed sheet. Then place a large bath towel over the plastic covering so the patient's skin does not directly touch the uncomfortable plastic lining.

2) Gently assist the patient so he is repositioned lower in the bed.

3) Place a pillow under his shoulders so his head is slightly raised.

4) Place a basin under his head. Be sure his neck is not leaning uncomfortably on the edge of the basin.

5) Using a pitcher, pour several cups of warm water over the patient's hair so it becomes wet. All water should be contained within the basin. Shampoo hair. Rinse with warm water using the pitcher. Towel dry. A blow dryer may be used to avoid a chill, especially if the weather is cold.

Changing a Bottom Sheet on an Occupied Bed

Even if your patient is unable to get out of bed, you can still change the bottom sheet of his bed without any discomfort to him. Ideally, sheets (bottom and top) should be changed every day and straightened often during the day as needed. If the sheets become soiled, then, of course, you will need to change them more often.

1) "Log roll" the patient toward you so she is in a side-lying position, close to the edge of the bed. She should be facing you. If she is in a hospital bed, raise the side rails for protection. If not, position yourself so she cannot fall out of bed.

2) Roll one half of the soiled bottom sheet lengthwise so it gathers in the middle of the bed.

3) Roll a clean bottom sheet lengthwise and place one half of it where the soiled one had been with the remainder of the clean sheet rolled in the center of the bed next to the rolled soiled one.

4) "Log roll" the patient onto the clean half of the bed. Remove the soiled sheet. While the patient remains in a side-lying position facing the opposite direction from where you are standing, unroll the remainder of the clean sheet and tuck it in. The bottom sheet should be stretched tightly so wrinkles in the sheet do not irritate the patient's fragile skin.

5) Reposition your patient with pillows for comfort.

Using a Draw Sheet

A draw sheet is placed in between the patient and the bottom sheet. Using a draw sheet will assist you in turning and lifting your patient in bed. It is more comfortable for your patient to be lifted and repositioned using a draw sheet and will help you, the caregiver, to avoid back strain.

1) Fold a flat sheet in half lengthwise and place on the bed crosswise. It should extend from the patient's shoulders to his knees. (Some

caregivers prefer that it extend from the patient's head to his knees.) Tuck in the extra long edges so they do not hang down the sides of the bed. A draw sheet should fit tightly over the bottom sheet.

2) When turning the patient to a side-lying position, simply undo the end of the draw sheet opposite to the side of the bed in which you want your patient to be moved.

3) Walk around to the other side of the bed, lean forward and take hold of the loosened end of the draw sheet. Use the draw sheet to "log roll" your patient toward you to a side-lying position. Again, stretch the draw sheet tightly and tuck under the mattress.

4) Two caregivers are required to lift your patient up in bed using the draw sheet. Patients who are bedridden tend to slide down in the bed as the day goes on. This can become uncomfortable, especially if the patient's feet are simply hanging off the end of the bed. (This can create a painful condition in bedridden patients, sometimes referred to as "foot drop." Immobility and poor positioning cause the muscles in the feet to stretch forward.) Several times a day, your patient may require a helpful "boost" so his head remains at the top of the bed and his feet do not hang off the bottom edge. (It is recommended to place a rolled pillow or blanket at the foot of the bed to help avoid "foot drop" and also to help keep the patient from sliding down the bed.) To reposition your patient up in bed, undo both ends of the draw sheet. Each caregiver holds on to an end and, on the count of three, gently lifts the patient up in bed. Avoid sliding the patient in bed to avoid skin abrasions caused by friction. Again, stretch both ends of the draw sheet and tuck them tightly under the mattress.

Preventing Decubitus Ulcers (Pressure Sores)

A decubitus ulcer, or pressure sore, is a break in the skin and underlying tissue caused by pressure or friction. If your patient is repositioned at least every two hours round the clock, the skin is kept clean and moisturized, and bony prominences are padded with soft pillows, there should be no reason why she should develop pressure ulcers. However, as body systems begin to fail and circulation becomes impaired, your task of preventing skin breakdown will be greatly challenged. Generalized poor health, muscle wasting, poor healing, anemia, incontinence, and poor nutritional intake combined with immobility present a challenge for the caregiver in terms of preventing skin breakdown. Obese patients are at risk because they exert greater pressure on the body as a whole and emaciated patients are at risk because bony prominences are not cushioned by fatty tissue.

In any terminally ill patient, skin can become so fragile that, as previously stated, a wrinkled bed sheet can present problems. In addition, friction rubs on bed sheets can open delicate skin. Oxygen tubing that is mistakenly left under a patient's arm or back can cause an indentation in poorly circulating tissue and can lead to an opening in the skin. If your patient has an indwelling urinary catheter in place, be sure to position the tubing so it is not under the patient. I had a patient whose primary caregiver had not noticed that the catheter tubing was under the patient's upper thigh for more than six hours. (Obviously, the patient had not been repositioned at least every two hours as recommended.) By the time I arrived at the home as a visiting nurse, pressure from the tubing had already caused the skin to open and bleed. Skin breakdown can occur that quickly. Often caregivers are reluctant to "disturb" their resting patient, but bedsores will ultimately be much more disturbing. Reposition! Reposition! Reposition!

Pressure sores occur mostly on the parts of the body that bear the most body weight. Consequently, bony prominences, such as the back of the head, shoulder blades, elbows, knees, hips, spine (especially the sacrum and coccyx), buttocks, ankles, and heels are especially vulnerable.

Decubitus ulcers are classified into four stages. Careful inspection of the skin is required at least once or twice daily. A good time to do this is while giving a bed bath or changing bedclothes. Any reddened area should immediately be brought to the attention of the hospice nurse or physician. In this way, a Stage 1 pressure sore can be treated early, preventing further complications and advanced staging.

> **Stage 1:** A specific area of skin appears pink or red. (It can be smaller than the circumference of a dime). The skin is unbroken, but there is superficial capillary damage. When pressed with a finger, the skin blanches (whitens), lasting up to 15 minutes after the pressure is

released. The skin area may feel warm to the touch. Patients often complain that the area is painful. If left untreated, Stage 1 pressure sores become deep and more difficult to heal.

Stage 2: There is an opening in the skin that appears cracked, broken, or blistered. The surrounding area is red. A small amount of drainage may be noted.

Stage 3: The skin is broken, with deep tissue involvement. There is usually a considerable amount of foul-smelling drainage.

Stage 4: The skin is broken, with deep tissue involvement that can include muscle. The cavity is deep and can expose bone. The wound may be small or larger than a fist. There is usually blackish, necrotic tissue visible within the cavity. It is foul-smelling, with a considerable amount of drainage.

What can be Done to Avoid Pressure Sores?

Back to Basics

- Use a draw sheet to lift and reposition the patient. Never pull the patient up in bed, as the friction and shearing will cause skin and capillary damage. Reposition the patient at least every two hours. Have plenty of soft pillows with clean pillowcases on hand. If in a side-lying position, bend the patient's knees and place a pillow between them so the sides of his knees are not rubbing together. Place a pillow under the head and dependent shoulder. Place a pillow between the ankles as well. Without exhausting the patient, try various positions and pillow placement until he is comfortable and free from pressure on bony prominences.

- If the patient is able to sit in a chair, pad the bottom, back and arms of the chair with soft pillows or other cushions.

- Perform passive range of motion exercise on the patient. Whether the patient is conscious or unconscious, every two hours gently bend arms inward and straighten them again, move each finger in toward the palms, rotate wrists, bend legs and straighten them again, rotate feet at the ankles, wiggle each toe. This will increase circulation as well as prevent muscle and joint stiffness. Gently support the head while turning it from side to side. Immobility can cause tremendous stiffness and discomfort in the neck.

- Consider using a foam "egg-crate" mattress over the existing mattress. (Always cover this with a bed sheet so the foam does not irritate the skin.) Foam "egg-crate" mattresses are not expensive and can be purchased at most department stores. They provide a little extra cushioning and allow more air to circulate under and around the skin. If the patient is on a home hospice program, the hospice may provide one or may suggest another type of specialty mattress, such as an air mattress, to prevent or treat existing pressure sores.

- Protective heel pads are available at most medical supply stores or may be provided by your hospice nurse. They are usually made from thick padded cotton. Many are machine washable. Similar protective pads are available for elbows as well. Heels are especially vulnerable to pressure sores. Check the bottom of your patient's heels often for redness or opening in the skin. Keep them moisturized and protected from dry and cracking skin. If heel pads are unavailable, you can improvise by wrapping a soft, thick piece of material under and around the patient's heel and securing it on the top of the foot with a small piece of Velcro-like material. Be sure it is not too tight so circulation is not impaired. Unless it is contraindicated, place a soft pillow under the patient's calves when he is resting on his back so his heels are lifted one or two inches off the mattress and are relieved of pressure.

- Keep the bed clean with sheets tucked in tightly to avoid wrinkles against fragile skin.

- Keep your patient's skin clean and dry. Offer gentle back rubs with a moisturizing lotion to improve circulation and provide comfort. Moisturize bony areas such as inner ankles, shoulder blades, and knees.

- Bacteria will increase the risk of skin breakdown and infection. If your patient is incontinent of bladder and/or bowel, provide excellent cleansing and skin care, including liberal application of a moisture barrier cream.

- If nutritional intake is poor, provide daily doses of vitamin C to maintain collagen and connective tissue in the skin. Zinc gluconate tablets can be helpful as well for healing skin.

Personal care will take many forms and can include such simple acts as placing a cool cloth on a patient's forehead or lightly stroking her arm for reassurance. It is intimate and should be performed with the utmost regard for your patient's dignity. Though it is often nonverbal, if done correctly it will convey to your patient an important message of caring and respect.

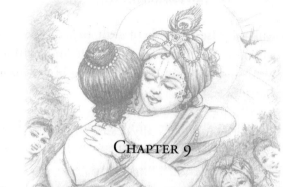

CHAPTER 9

Complementary Therapies for Comfort Care

This chapter addresses some complementary therapies that can be implemented in conjunction with the current medical regimen of the terminally ill patient. Whether the patient prefers the use of conventional allopathic medicine (see Chapter 7) or alternative treatments, such as homeopathic, herbal, or Ayurvedic medicine, the pain that every terminally ill patient is burdened with should be relieved so the remainder of his days can be spent in peaceful meditation on the lotus feet of the Lord.

After consulting with the patient's physician or hospice nurse to be sure there are no contraindications, the following complementary therapies can be tried and, if effective, can be administered alongside current medical treatment to provide additional relief from various discomforts. The complementary therapies discussed below should never be considered as a replacement for medications to relieve the severe pain experienced in a terminal illness.

Relaxation Techniques

Relaxation techniques can reduce the anxiety associated with chronic pain and assist the patient in coping with the stressors associated with a poor prognosis. When successful, relaxation techniques can relieve physical signs of anxiety, such as a rapid heartbeat and increased respirations. Two types of relaxation therapies, guided imagery and music therapy, follow.

Guided Imagery

Tibetan monks have long used guided imagery as a means of healing by visualizing the Buddha curing diseases. Historically, people in various cultures have found ways to alter their state of consciousness to enhance their inner lives and as a means to physically, emotionally, and spiritually heal.

At present, guided imagery is used in many therapeutic settings to relieve anxiety, depression, headache, insomnia, and to treat symptoms often exhibited in cancer patients, such as nausea and vomiting, anorexia, digestive disorders, and itching (often a side effect of pain medications). Guided imagery can assist a patient to better cope with pain and alleviate nausea in chemotherapy patients. It utilizes the power of the mind to promote tranquility and a sense of general well being. It has been effective in decreasing anxiety in patients prior to surgical procedures and to hasten postoperative recovery. Guided imagery can lower blood pressure and decrease heart rate. It has been documented to affect brain wave activity, skin temperature, and vascular constriction. In a hospice setting, it is often used by practitioners to relax patients and to decrease symptoms such as nausea and headache.

Certified practitioners of guided imagery are those who have completed an extensive program of course work, although many hospice nurses successfully perform some form of guided imagery as a means of calming their patients. As with other relaxation techniques, guided imagery should complement—never replace—other therapies instituted by the patient's physician.

Guided imagery is based on the principle that images created in the mind can be almost as real as actual, external events. It is the use of a person's imagination to create mental images that can involve all of the senses. The more vividly someone is able to imagine a scene, called image generation, the more receptive that person will be to guided imagery. An even more important skill required by the patient is the ability to become absorbed in sensory or imaginative experiences. This trait is called absorption. People with powerful imaginations have the ability to connect so intensely with a particular mental image that they are able to experience smells, tastes, sounds, and tactile sensations. During a guided imagery exercise, the patient actually senses the image, not just visualizes it. Music can sometimes increase the effects of imagery as can a scent that may elicit a specific memory. In addition, imagery combined with therapeutic massage and rhythmic breathing may be helpful to relax your patient. Proponents of guided imagery maintain that there are many correct ways to perform this mind-body intervention and that the more it is practiced, the more the practitioner and patient will benefit.

Basically, there are three types of guided imagery. The first type, **Stress Reduction and Relaxation Guided Imagery**, is the one practiced by most nurses unless they have more in-depth training. It is used to decrease generalized anxiety, caused by the anticipation of a medical procedure, pain reduction, nausea, insomnia, and itchiness.

The second type of guided imagery, called **Directed-Active Guided Imagery**, is based on the idea that the imagination speaks in pictures, symbols, and metaphors. The practitioner must understand the language of the unconscious mind and adapt metaphors and create pictures and symbols to help with the specific needs of the patient. For example, imagining yourself crossing a bridge can symbolize leaving something behind, perhaps something unpleasant, and entering a new beginning in one's life.

The third type of guided imagery is called **Insight-Oriented Guided Imagery**. Briefly, this involves the patient interacting with an imaginary "wise" personality as directed by the person leading the guided imagery session. The patient may ask this "wise" person what is needed to feel better or how he can better cope with his illness. Often the guide may encourage the patient to reenter a dream he had while sleeping to further explore its meaning.

Whatever type of guided imagery you will be performing, plan sufficient time for the guided imagery therapy session and be sure there will be no interruptions. The first type of imagery, used for stress reduction and relaxation, can take one to two minutes or up to twenty minutes or longer. Create a peaceful atmosphere for the patient by dimming bright lights and reducing environmental noise as much as possible. Background sound vibration can include Srila Prabhupada's *japa* meditation tape or a soft *bhajan*. If the patient prefers, the room can remain silent except for your calming voice. Assist the patient into a comfortable position. Explain that when the first phase is completed, her entire body should feel relaxed and her mind calm. This exercise works best when the patient's eyes are closed. Exact wording and sequence of coaching can be modified according to personal preference and the consciousness of your patient. The caregiver should speak in a soft, monotone voice to induce a sense of calm.

The following exercise combines a form of rhythmic breathing along with guided imagery, but rhythmic breathing does not have to be included if it causes any distress for your patient. If the patient exhibits any shortness of breath related to anxiety, it would be beneficial to "talk him down" (so to speak) by helping him to slow each breath. Sit close to your patient. While directly facing him, slowly breathe in and out, encouraging him to follow your rhythm. Pursed lip breathing, as previously described, may be helpful. If the patient's shortness of breath or difficult respirations are attributed to his disease process, it may not be possible to have him participate in the rhythmic breathing portion of this exercise. However, guided imagery without rhythmic breathing may relax him enough to improve any shortness of breath.

Using a calm, quiet tone, instruct the patient as follows:

- Inhale slowly. While you exhale, relax your feet, first the right foot and then the left. Slowly breathe in and out as you feel your toes and ankles relax. With each breath, breathe calmness in and anxiety out.

- Now concentrate on releasing any tension in the back of your calves, first the right calf and then the left. As you breathe in and out, you will feel your feet and calves relax.

- Inhale slowly. Exhale slowly while you breathe out any tension and worry. Now release any tightness in your thighs. The muscles in your legs are relaxed and you are beginning to feel calm.

- Now feel the muscles release in your abdomen.

- Slowly breathe in and out and feel your chest rise and fall with each breath.

- Let go of any tension you are holding in your fingers, your hands, your wrists, and your arms. Relax your shoulders. Allow your arms to sink deeply into the bed.

- Take a slow, deep breath and, while you exhale, feel all of the tension release from your neck. If your jaw is clenched, release it now. Relax the muscles in your face as you slowly exhale.

- Now feel the relaxation throughout your whole body, from your toes to the top of your head. Continue to breathe slowly, in and out, as your entire body goes limp and you feel a tremendous release of stress. Your whole body is calm and peaceful for the next part of your journey.

During the next phase, ask your patient to go to a place where she feels safe, warm, and tranquil. This place will differ for each patient. Perhaps it will be at a holy place in India where she once traveled during healthier days. Perhaps it will be on a beach or on a mountain or in a field of tall grass on a farm. Wherever her "safe place" may be, allow her to spend as much time there as she wishes. Encourage her to notice the details around her, such as the sounds, the smells, or the warmth of the sun on her face. Tell her that when she is ready to leave, she can picture herself walking away from that peaceful place while taking the tranquility with her. Ask her to open her eyes and to slowly become aware of her external environment.

If the patient agrees, this exercise can be modified to increase his meditation on the Deity of the Lord. Ask him which Deities he would like to visit. It would be helpful if you had a picture of Their Lordships during this exercise. Unless contraindicated because of the use of oxygen equipment or for medical reasons such as respiratory difficulty, nausea, or other medical conditions, incense or a scented candle can be lit beforehand to engage his sense of smell and elicit memories of devotional service. His sense of hearing can be engaged by playing a soft chanting recording in the background. He will also hear your calming voice throughout the exercise. After assisting your patient into a comfortable position and performing the initial breathing and relaxation exercise as described above, encourage him to visualize himself entering a temple, paying obeisances, and then taking *darshan* of the Deities. Using the picture of the Deities, start with the lotus feet of the Lord and describe in detail what is seen. Can he see the *tulasi* leaves placed on the Lord's moonlike toes? What is the Lord wearing? Describe the color of His *dhoti*, the brilliance of His jewels, and the opulence of His crown. Describe in which direction the Lord's peacock feather is facing. Describe the alternating colors and sweet fragrance of the Lord's flower garland. Is Krishna's flute gold or silver? Include vivid descriptions of Tulasi Devi on the altar. What color is her skirt? How large are her leaves and *manjaris*? What other Deities are on the altar? Describe the spotless marble on the steps of the altar and its scent of eucalyptus. Allow the patient to take *darshan* of the Deities as long as he wishes. Softly remind him that *darshan* sees both ways. He is happy to see the Lord, and the Lord is even happier that His dear devotee has come to visit Him. Near the altar, there is a bright silver tray piled with multicolored flower petals. Pick up a handful of petals and offer them at the Lord's lotus feet. Tell him that when he is ready to leave, visualize offering obeisances and exiting the temple. Remind him to take with him the tranquility of being in the presence of the Lord. Softly remind him that the Deities are all-pervading and remain with him always. Lord Krishna is in his heart. Ask him to open his eyes and to slowly become aware of his external environment.

This exercise can be modified to include visualizing a favorite place of pilgrimage, or rendering a much-loved devotional service that the patient is now physically incapable of performing, or meditating on attending a favorite festival such as *Rathayatra* or *Govardhan Puja*. It is up to the patient to choose her place and activity for obtaining peace. For your patient, an imaginary walk along a peaceful beach while overlooking the ocean waves, or sitting in a meadow filled with wild flowers, or a hike to a favorite mountain may prove relaxing. Whichever image you guide your patient to visualize, this technique takes time, but its benefits will be well worth it.

Music Therapy

Historically, music therapy dates back to Pythagoras, who taught that singing and playing musical instruments could counteract negative emotions. Today many hospitals and hospice programs utilize music therapy to reduce anxiety in children, adolescents, and adults. It has been successfully used to communicate with disoriented patients afflicted with Alzheimer's disease as well as aiding in the rehabilitation of stroke patients. Music therapy is also used in rehabilitation facilities when working with persons with brain injuries. It has been said to reduce the stress associated with labor and childbirth. In addition, studies conclude that meaningful music can have a positive effect on patients suffering from depression and other psychiatric disorders. Many proponents of music therapy suggest that musical sound vibration, when used for relaxation and healing, affects the brain in such a way as to decrease rapid heart rate, reduce blood pressure, slow breathing, reduce muscle tension, aid in digestion, and induce sleep. In general, music is said to be therapeutically calming when it is slower than the patient's pulse or slower than 60 beats per minute.

As Vaishnavas, we understand the importance of transcendental sound vibration to calm the mind and body and to awaken our spiritual consciousness. In a letter I received from His Divine Grace Srila Prabhupada, dated August 29, 1973, Srila Prabhupada writes:

> The chanting (of the Hare Krishna *mantra*) is a process of purification. Just like we use soap to cleanse the body—this is material—but the chanting is a spiritual cleansing. The three stages of cleansing are first to clean the mirror of the mind... Due to long-term association, the mind absorbed in material things has become contaminated, or dirty. The chanting process purifies the mind. Then the next stage, when the mind is cleansed, one becomes free from the symptoms of material existence. Material existence means to be always hankering and lamenting: 'I must have a new automobile, I must have more money, I must have a good wife, I must have this, I must have that.' Then when I have the thing, I lament, 'I have lost my wife, I have lost my money, I have lost my car,' simply lamenting. So, the second stage is to be free from this anxiety. The third stage is, 'He never laments nor desires to have anything. He is equally disposed to every living entity. In that state he attains pure devotional service unto me.' (*Bhagavad-gita As It Is*, 18.54) The next verse continues, 'And when one is in full consciousness of the Supreme Lord, by such devotion he can enter into the kingdom of God.' It is further stated in the *Gita* that when one is so situated even in the midst of greatest danger he is not disturbed. In other words, when one has achieved perfection in chanting the Holy Name of God, he is always joyful. Even death does not disturb him, what to speak of other things. The conclusion is that one should learn the art of chanting the Holy Name of Krishna 24 hours a day and that alone is the remedy for all problems of material existence...So I cannot give you any better advice. Simply chant Hare Krishna and everything will be all right.

We have been blessed with this knowledge, and as caregivers we can give our patients no better music therapy for true peace than the chanting of the Hare Krishna mantra and the many wonderful devotional songs written by the great *acharyas*. According to the patient's physical and mental condition, as well as his wishes, a soft *japa* or *bhajan* tape can be played or devotees can visit for soft chanting or a quiet *bhajan*. Depending on how he feels, the patient may desire a more enthusiastic *kirtan* with *mrdanga* drum and *karatals*. Or perhaps he may prefer to simply chant *japa* alone or with one or two other devotees. In any case, be sure to give him a choice and to respect his wishes. Facilitating a Vaishnava's Krishna consciousness by providing "transcendental music therapy" is the greatest service you can render.

Aromatherapy

Aromatherapy is the therapeutic use of essential oils extracted from various plants. The flowers, leaves, stem, and roots from noted plants are used to promote relaxation and to provide relief from various mental and physical ailments. Aromatherapy is based on the principle that receptors in the nose convert scents to nerve impulses that are sent to the limbic system of the brain, where memory and mood are controlled. The brain then responds to a particular scent by associating it with past memories. The emotions that are evoked can affect blood pressure, heart rate, respirations, and the release of hormones, neurotransmitters, and endorphins. Even a long-forgotten smell can trigger powerful memories, either pleasant or unpleasant. If the scent is unfamiliar, then a new response and memory are created.

A scent can be either calming or energizing and stimulating. In addition, some essential oils possess antibacterial, antiseptic, and antiviral properties. In parts of Europe, aromatherapy has been used for many years during labor and delivery, not only to relax the mother but also to reduce fetal distress and to stabilize fetal heart rate. In fact, aromatherapy course work is mandatory in midwifery training in Germany.

During the past three decades, aromatherapy has become more popular in the United States as a complementary treatment that is used alongside traditional medicine. It is often used to relieve stress, anxiety, depression, and insomnia. Proponents use essential oils to help relieve headache, muscle and joint pain, digestive upset, nausea, premenstrual syndrome, some skin disorders, and chest and nasal congestion due to a cold or flu. Oils can be mixed with lotion or a carrier oil for massage, dabbed on a cloth for inhalation, added to bath water, used in vaporizers, placed in a bowl of hot water for steam inhalation, or placed in a basin of warm water for a relaxing footbath. It is important to purchase essential oils through a reputable company. Often, synthetic perfumes are sold as aromatherapy products, using the names "perfume oil," "botanical perfume," or "fragrance oil."

Aromatherapy should never be instituted without consulting your patient's physician or hospice nurse. It should never be used as a substitute for appropriate medical care. Use of some essential oils can be toxic to pregnant women or mothers who are breast-feeding. It is contraindicated in patients with conditions such as epilepsy, heart disease, diabetes, kidney or liver disorders, or patients with open wounds. Some essential oils, such as rosemary and eucalyptus, are toxic to infants and children under five years of age. It is recommended that a certified aromatherapist be consulted before using essential oils. Some hospice nurses are knowledgeable in this subject and may be able to recommend specific oils that would complement the patient's current medical regimen. Pure essential oils are highly concentrated and thorough knowledge of their use is vital.

Uses of pure essential oils differ, but they are so concentrated that basic guidelines include the following:

For massage: Dilute five drops of oil in 10 milliliters of lotion or carrier oil. Undiluted essential oil should never be applied directly to the skin. Keep oils away from eyes and mouth, but if the oils do come in contact with the patient's eyes, flush the eyes profusely with cool water and consult a medical practitioner if pain or burning persists.

For inhalation: Place only one drop of oil on a tissue or cloth. Place the tissue or cloth near the patient's nose, but not so close as to irritate mucous membranes.

For bath: Add six drops of oil to warm bath water. Assist the patient into the tub and ask her to gently inhale the vapors for 10-20 minutes or as tolerated. Please note that hot baths are not recommended during pregnancy or for patients with conditions such as multiple sclerosis, diabetes, or hyper- or hypo- blood pressure. Always assist your patient when getting out of a hot tub in case of dizziness or fainting.

For vaporizer: Fill the vaporizer up with water to ¾ full and add four drops of oil.

For footbath: Place six drops of oil in a basin of warm water. If the patient is in bed, assist him in bending his knees and place his feet in the basin for a few minutes. Dry the feet immediately after removing them from the water.

For steam inhalation: Add eight drops to a bowl of hot water. Position the bowl near the patient so that when a large towel is placed over the patient's upper body and bowl of water, she will be able to inhale the vapors for a few minutes. *Caution*: If your patient is weak, drowsy, or disoriented, she may require assistance holding her head a sufficient distance away from the hot water so her face is not scalded.

In a hospice setting, if it is agreeable with the physician or hospice nurse, any of the above methods of aromatherapy could be helpful for relief of stress and various discomforts. If your patient is bed-ridden and it is medically appropriate, a warm footbath or gentle back rub using essential oil in lotion or carrier oil may be comforting. (See "Therapeutic Massage for the Terminally Ill Patient.") Essential oils may be used when giving a bed bath for relaxation and to relieve muscle soreness.

I know of some nurses working with patients with Alzheimer's disease who use aromatherapy at the end of the day when the sun is going down. Patients with Alzheimer's tend to exhibit increased agitation at sundown. (This is referred to as "Sundowner's Syndrome.") The nurses place a drop of oil meant for relaxation, such as Mandarin oil, on a cotton ball. They then attach the cotton ball to the lapel or collar of the patient's dress or jacket with a safety pin. (Some disoriented patients think it is a small flower and are pleased to wear it.) The cotton ball remains close enough to the patient's nose to provide a calming effect from the scent of the oil. This same principle can be applied in a hospice setting with patients who are experiencing end-stage anxiety.

The following list of essential oils is not meant to be all-inclusive, but may be helpful if appropriate for your patient's condition. Roman chamomile and lavender, when used as a complementary therapy with other treatments, have shown positive effects in relieving anxiety and generalized discomfort in some cancer patients in a hospice setting.

Some Suggested Essential Oils

Angelica Root Oil (*Angelica archangelica*) is extracted from the root, fruit, or seed of the plant. Its use dates back to at least the 14th and 15th centuries during the plagues and was used to ward off infection. It has a musky, pepper-like scent and is said to make a good expectorant, aid in digestion, relieve muscle discomfort, and help relieve coughs and colds. It is known to be a relaxant.

Angelica root oil can be mixed in carrier oil for massage, placed in baths for relaxation and to reduce muscle tension, placed in a bowl of hot water and its vapors inhaled to relieve congestion from a cough or cold, or placed on a warm cloth and used as a compress. A drop of angelica root oil on a tissue can help clear nasal congestion due to a cold.

Caution: Avoid sunlight after use or it may cause skin irritation. This oil is not to be used during pregnancy.

Avocado Oil (*Persea gratissima*) is extracted from the fruit of the tree. It is used for treating skin conditions such as eczema and sunburn. It may be helpful to patients with dry skin. It is used as a base, or carrier oil, for massage.

Basil Oil (*Ocimum basilicum*) is extracted from the flowering sweet basil plant. It is used for anxiety, insomnia, fatigue, headache, poor circulation, and muscle aches. Basil oil can be mixed in carrier oil or lotion for massage, placed in a bath to increase circulation and relieve aching muscles, or added to a bowl of hot water for inhalation. This oil can be dabbed on a tissue for inhalation or on a compress placed on the forehead to relieve a headache.

Caution: Basil oil is extremely potent and may cause skin irritation. It should never be used during pregnancy.

Clove Oil (*Eugenia carophyllata*) is extracted by steam distillation from the flowers. It is known for its antiseptic properties and also makes a good mosquito repellent. Clove oil is sometimes used in mouthwash. It has been traditionally used to relieve toothaches by rubbing the oil on gums.

This oil has a spicy, stimulating scent, but can also be warming and relaxing. In aromatherapy, it is helpful with generalized aches and pains, back pain, and is used as a muscle relaxant. It can be used for massage and in a warm bath to sooth and relax.

Caution: Clove oil must be very well diluted or skin irritation may occur. It should never be used during pregnancy.

Eucalyptus Oil (*Eucalyptus globules*) is extracted from the twigs and leaves of the Blue Gum tree. Historically, aborigines crushed the leaves of the tree to heal wounds and fight infections. Today, eucalyptus oil is used in many cough and cold remedies and is helpful as a decongestant and expectorant. It has antiseptic properties that kill airborne germs. It is used to relieve some symptoms of a cold, flu, or sinus infection and has been helpful in reducing nausea. When diluted properly, the essential oil also soothes muscle aches and aids in healing skin abrasions. It can be used for massage, in a soothing bath, as inhalation therapy when diluted in a bowl of hot water and used as a decongestant, dabbed on a warm compress and placed on the chest to clear congestion, and diluted in water as a disinfectant when cleansing the patient's room.

Caution: This oil is very strong and should be diluted well.

Lavender Oil (*Lavandula angustifolia*) is extracted from the leaves of the evergreen shrub and is often used to decrease tension, fatigue, and depression. It is helpful with some skin problems, in relieving generalized aches and pains, and has anti-inflammatory and antibacterial properties. It can relieve a headache, a toothache, and soothe stomach discomfort. Lavender oil is used for massage, warm baths, inhalation therapy, and compresses. When a few drops of lavender oil are placed in a hot bath, it produces drowsiness and decreased anxiety and stress. When placed in a cool bath, this oil refreshes and energizes and produces a feeling of well being.

Mandarin Oil (*Citrus reticulata*) is extracted from the peel of the ripe fruit of the citrus tree. In aromatherapy, it is used as a sedative and can help relieve headaches. It is also used as a digestive stimulant. It has a relaxing effect and can decrease stress, restlessness, and nervous tension. It can be helpful when a patient is feeling irritable. This oil is used for massage, baths, inhalation therapy, or can be dabbed on a tissue to decrease anxiety.

Caution: This oil should be used in moderation or it can cause skin irritation. Some patients experience photosensitivity (sensitivity to the sun or other ultraviolet light source) after use and should be cautioned to stay out of the sun immediately after use of this oil.

Peppermint Oil (*Mentha piperita*) is extracted from fresh or semi-dried leaves and flowers of the herb. Historically, it has been found in Egyptian tombs dating back to 1000 BC. It has long been known for its antibacterial and antiviral properties. Today, peppermint oil is used to invigorate, refresh, and cool. It is used to relieve headaches, mental fatigue, muscle aches, and nausea. It is also used to stimulate digestion. A few drops diluted in warm water can provide a refreshing footbath for your patient. Peppermint oil is diluted and used for massage, baths, inhalation therapy, and on compresses. A drop of oil on a tissue may relieve nausea.

Caution: Peppermint oil is very potent and should be used in moderation. Dilute carefully. Since it can act as a stimulant, it should never be used before going to sleep.

Sandalwood Mysore Oil (*Santalum album*) is extracted from the roots and wood of the tree. Most sandalwood essential oil comes from India. This oil is an antiseptic and is used as an astringent. It has a sedative effect and is therefore helpful in reducing stress, tension, insomnia, and depression. It is often used as an expectorant for coughs and colds or diluted in carrier oil and used as a moisturizer for dry skin. Diluted oil can be used for massage, baths, inhalation therapy for relief of congestion, and compresses to reduce anxiety and soothe aching muscles and joints.

Roman Chamomile Oil (*Anthemis nobilis*) is extracted from freshly-dried flowers. The essential oil contains azulene, a natural anti-inflammatory. It is used for stress, insomnia, headaches, skin rashes, burns, cuts, insect bites, toothaches, and menstrual and menopausal ailments. It is used for massage, baths, inhalation therapy, and compresses for headaches and menstrual discomfort.

Geranium Oil (*Pelargonium graveolens*) is extracted from the flowers, stalks, and leaves of the shrub. It has a sweet, mint-like scent that is used as a sedative. Geranium oil has antiviral and antifungal properties. It is diluted with a carrier oil or lotion to relieve dry, flaky skin. It can be used in massage, baths, inhalation therapy, or compresses. In a hot bath, this oil is relaxing; in cool water it is stimulating and energizing.

For thousands of years, essential oils have been used to soothe the mind, body, and spirit. As previously stated, the above list is not meant to be all-inclusive. There are many more essential oils that may be appropriate for your hospice patient, and research into their healing properties may be of value.

Herbal Therapy

Following is a list of some of the more popular herbs along with usages and cautions. There are many healing herbs for a variety of symptoms. Neither the list of herbs nor the usages stated for each are intended to be all-inclusive. Please remember that even "natural" remedies can have negative effects or toxic levels if taken incorrectly or in the wrong combination. They can also have adverse interactions with allopathic medications or other medical therapies your patient may be using. Further, current laws in the United States allow herbal products to be regulated as if they were food and not medications. Therefore, the Food and Drug Administration (FDA) cannot apply the same standards for their production as with prescriptions or over-the-counter medicines. Always consult with a licensed herbalist for correct dosages and with your patient's medical doctor before starting any herbal therapy. Please be aware that many herbal tinctures are made with alcohol to extract the medicinal ingredients and to act as a preservative.

One more word of caution: Although this is a book for the care of hospice patients, I would like to mention, for the sake of other readers, that many herbs are contraindicated during pregnancy due to their stimulating effect on the uterus. If an incorrect herb is taken at this time, it could cause premature delivery, which could cause a host of complications for the newborn.

Cranberry: Also called *Vaccinium macrocarpon*, this herb is useful in fighting urinary tract infections. The berry part of the shrub is used and comes in capsule or juice form. It is sometimes difficult to purchase 100% pure cranberry juice as it is often mixed with other fruit juices, water, and sugar. There are no adverse reactions reported concerning this commonly used herb.

Echinacea: Native Americans originally used echinacea, also known as "purple coneflower," for fevers, snake bites, and wounds. Over the last fifty years, echinacea has become well known for its antibacterial, antiviral, and antifungal properties. It is frequently used for colds, flu, and upper respiratory infections. It can also be used as a wash for infected wounds and as a gargle for sore throats. The part of the plant most commonly used is the root, which can be powdered and placed into capsules.

High dosages may cause dizziness and nausea. There are also controversial findings that echinacea may exacerbate certain conditions such as HIV, AIDS, tuberculosis, and multiple sclerosis. Echinacea should not be taken with drugs that are toxic to the liver such as some steroids (e.g., amiodarone, methotrexate, ketoconazole) as usage of this herb, even if taken alone for more than eight weeks, could cause hepatoxicity (liver toxicity).

Feverfew: Feverfew, also known as featherfew, has a long history of use for fever reduction and nausea. It was also applied externally for headaches. Recently, feverfew has become popular for the management and prevention of migraine headaches. It is believed that it may also lower blood pressure as well as ease the pain of chronic inflammation, as in arthritis.

Aerial (above ground) parts of the feverfew plant are used. The fresh leaves can be used to make an infusion (placing leaves in a container, pouring hot water over them, and steeping for ten minutes) or the leaves and flowers may be dried and put into capsules.

Because feverfew decreases blood clotting, it should not be taken after surgery or used by patients who are on blood-thinning drugs such as aspirin. Chewing the fresh leaves may cause mouth ulcers. If more than the recommended dosage is taken, this herb could cause gastrointestinal upset or nervousness. Feverfew is contraindicated in patients allergic to ragweed.

Ginkgo Biloba: The ginkgo tree is also known as the maidenhair tree. Ginkgo is used for circulatory diseases, and in particular for improving blood flow to the brain. This herb is said to benefit some patients with Alzheimer's disease, atherosclerosis (hardening or narrowing of the arteries), stroke, congestive heart failure, depression, diabetes, and multiple sclerosis. It has also been used for varicose veins, hemorrhoids, leg ulcers, tinnitus, and headaches caused by constriction of blood vessels.

Fresh leaves from the ginkgo tree are used for fluid extracts (a commercial product made to pharmaceutical specifications with increased strength of the herbal mixture), tinctures, and infusions, or the dried leaves for capsules. The seeds are used for decoctions.

Taking more than the stated dose can lead to headaches, skin disorders, or stomach upset. Gingko should not be taken with anticlotting medications, as this herb may inhibit blood clotting and cause bleeding.

Ginseng Root: Ginseng is a slow-growing plant that has been widely used in China for over five thousand years. The genus name *Panax* is Greek and literally means "cure-all." Historically, this root has been used as an aid during convalescence, to build resistance to illnesses, and to promote health and longevity. The use of multivitamins in the West is somewhat equivalent to the traditional use of ginseng root in Asia. There are three types of ginseng: Asian (the most well-known), Siberian, and American.

Ginseng is among the most studied of all medicinal herbs and is used for combating exhaustion, increasing concentration, stimulating the immune system, regulating levels of blood sugar and cholesterol, decreasing depression, and enhancing mood. Particular illnesses this herb might help include Alzheimer's, atherosclerosis, chronic fatigue syndrome, and flu.

The root of the ginseng plant is used for medicinal purposes. The whole root is often used in decoctions or tinctures or it is powdered and used in tablets or capsules.

Ginseng should be avoided by people with high blood pressure and should not be taken with stimulants such as caffeine. The World Health Organization (WHO) has cited two cases of adverse interaction between ginseng and the MAO inhibitor phenelzine (Nardil). Because it can thin the blood, it should not be taken with cardiac medications or with medication taken for diabetes. Ginseng should also be avoided by anyone who is pregnant as it could adversely affect the fetus. In rare occurrences it has caused overstimulation and insomnia.

Goldenseal: Goldenseal, or *Hydrastis canadensis*, was traditionally used by Native Americans for a variety of ailments including indigestion, fever, whooping cough, liver or heart problems, and gastric disorders.

Today, goldenseal is often used for colds and flu, especially in combination with echinacea. It is also said to strengthen the immune system, promote the functioning capacity of many of the body organs, and act as an antibacterial and antiviral agent. Diluted, it is sometimes used as an eyewash for conjunctivitis or as a mouthwash and gargle for gum disease, mouth ulcers, and sore throats.

Patients with high blood pressure should not take goldenseal. In addition, this herb may decrease the effects of anticlotting medications. Eating the fresh plant can cause mouth ulcers. High doses of goldenseal can cause gastrointestinal distress.

Kava Kava: Kava kava, or *Piper methysticum*, is a member of the pepper family and a popular herb in the South Pacific. It is used there for ceremonial purposes, including welcoming important guests.

This herb is most widely known for its relaxing qualities and is often used to reduce stress, restlessness, and nervous anxiety. Kava kava is also used as a muscle relaxant and for some of the symptoms associated with menopause, such as depressive moods, irritability, and hot flushes.

Continuous and/or large dosages of this herb can cause a temporary yellow coloring of the hair, skin, and nails. A few rare cases of allergic skin reactions have been noted. Patients who are taking barbiturates, antidepressants, or antianxiety medications should not take kava kava, as it can increase their effects. This herb increases sedation and when taken in combination with these medications can lead to coma.

Licorice Root: Licorice root, or *Glycyrrhiza glabra*, has been therapeutically used for thousands of years both in the West and in the East for a variety of symptoms. The ancient Greeks used licorice root as an expectorant, and it has been used in traditional Chinese medicine as an antiarrhythmic in cardiac patients. Much research has been done on this root, and it is widely used both medicinally and for flavoring.

Licorice is used for lowering blood cholesterol. In addition, it soothes gastric and duodenal ulcers, chronic gastritis pain, epigastric bloating, and the pain of rheumatism and arthritis. It is still used as an expectorant and as an anti-inflammatory agent. Licorice has also been used for herpes simplex, hypoglycemia, indigestion, some infections, and menopausal symptoms.

Patients with high blood pressure should avoid the use of licorice because it can cause sodium and fluid retention. It is also contraindicated with severe kidney insufficiency, liver disorders, hypokalemia (low potassium levels), and tachycardia (rapid heart rate). Licorice should not be taken with certain diuretics because it can cause further potassium loss. Increased sensitivity to the cardiac medication digitalis can occur when combined with this herb.

Toxic effects from overdose of licorice root may include weakness and lethargy, dulled reflexes, and high blood pressure.

Psyllium Seed: Blonde psyllium seed, obtained from *Plantago ovata*, is native to Iran and India; black psyllium seed, obtained from *Plantago afra*, is native to western Asia, northern Africa, and the western Mediterranean area. Both are now extensively cultivated in other countries. Psyllium is widely used for chronic constipation, irritable bowel syndrome, and increased cholesterol.

This herb should not be used by patients who have stenosis (narrowing) of the gastrointestinal tract, bowel obstruction, or poorly controlled diabetes. Absorption of other medications taken at the same time may be delayed.

St. John's Wort: Medicinal use of St. John's wort, or *Hypericum perforatum*, dates back to ancient Greece, where it was documented by herbalists for its therapeutic applications as a diuretic and for treatment of neuralgic conditions (nerve pain).

Today St. John's wort is most widely known for its antidepressant properties. It is also used to treat anxiety. Applied externally, this herb has been used to treat sprains, bruises, and wounds because of its anti-inflammatory effects.

The aerial parts of the St. John's wort plant are used. The leaves, stems, and flowers are used for infusions, tinctures, and washes (infusions or diluted tinctures used to bathe wounds, ulcers, or other skin conditions). The flowering tops are used to make infused oil (active plant ingredients extracted in oil) and cream, which are used externally.

It is generally believed that St. John's wort should not be taken with MAO inhibitor antidepressants. If higher than recommended doses are taken, this herb may cause photosensitivity, especially in fair-skinned individuals. Rash, severe burning, and skin blisters have been reported in those with photosensitivity. According to how it is processed, this herb may sometimes inhibit iron absorption.

Valerian Root: Valerian root, or *Valeriana officinalis*, has been used for at least two thousand years, but its responsible components and their modes of action are not completely understood. Sometimes referred to as "nature's tranquilizer," it is now primarily used to relieve nervous tension, anxiety, and insomnia. It is also used for healing wounds and ulcers, digestive problems, and dysmenorrhea (painful menstruation). It can be topically applied for muscle cramps. Valerian can be used alone, but is often combined in a tea with other herbs for relaxation.

The roots of the valerian plant are used to make infusions, tinctures, maceration (the process of softening by soaking the herb in cool fluid) soaks, compress soaks, and washes.

It is recommended that valerian not be taken for more than two to three weeks without a break as it may cause headaches and/or heart palpitations. This herb should not be taken with barbiturates, sleep-inducing drugs, certain antidepressants, or antihistamines, as it increases drowsiness.

Cutaneous Stimulation: Application of Heat and/or Cold for Pain Management

In some circumstances, applying external heat compresses and/or cold packs may decrease intensity of pain. At the very least, it can provide a distraction for your patient so his pain is more tolerable. Again, these methods should never be used as a substitute for analgesics or to increase the interval between doses of medication. After each application of heat and/or cold, ask the patient to evaluate its effectiveness so treatments can be continued or modified as needed. As with analgesics, noninvasive pain relief therapy is most effective when applied before the patient's pain is severe.

Thermotherapy (Heat Therapy)

External application of heat works by dilating the blood vessels so circulation to a particular area is increased. When blood circulation is increased to muscles, pain is often reduced. Applications of superficial heat may increase oxygen and nutrient delivery to damaged tissue and decrease joint stiffness. An electric heating pad (moist or dry), hot water bottle, or warm compress can be applied directly over the area of pain, or next to, above, or below the area of pain as tolerated. Generally, it is believed that moist heat is more effective than dry heat. Electric heating pads should always be properly covered with a cloth or towel and hot water bottles should be wrapped in a towel as well. More towels may be needed if the patient has decreased skin sensation. Heat should never be applied to skin that has been exposed to radiation treatment. During heat applications, be sure to check the skin frequently to ensure that the patient's skin is not reddened, burned, or blistered. This is especially important if the patient is confused, nonverbal, or unconscious.

Cryotherapy (Cold Therapy)

Cold therapy, such as the application of a cool compress, ice pack, or reusable gel pack, causes blood vessels to constrict, thus decreasing circulation to the area of treatment. Vasoconstriction helps to reduce inflammation and swelling which will often decrease a patient's pain. Cold packs also relieve headaches and joint pain caused by immobility, as well as muscle sprain or spasm. To be sure the intensity of the cold therapy is tolerable, it is recommended to place crushed ice in a well-sealed plastic bag and then wrap the bag in a towel or pillowcase. Ice packs should be flexible to conform to the patient's body contour. The patient should be kept warm with sufficient blankets during cold therapy so she does not develop a chill. The application of cold therapy should be less than that of heat therapy (less than 15 minutes). As with heat therapy, cold therapy should never be applied to skin that has been exposed to radiation therapy. Similarly, it is not recommended for application to areas with poor blood supply.

Ice Massage

A small paper cup can be completely filled with water and placed in a freezer until solid. The ice will freeze slightly above the rim of the cup and will provide a smooth surface for a comfortable massage. Place towels on both sides of the patient to catch any melting ice during the treatment. Apply the "ice massager" directly to the skin over soft tissue using small, circular motions. This should be done for approximately 5-10 minutes or as tolerated by the patient. Ice massage should be stopped when the patient feels the area has become numb. Exposing only the area being treated, be sure the patient is sufficiently covered with blankets during an ice massage.

Contrast Therapy

Alternating applications of heat and cold every few minutes to an affected area is known as contrast therapy. Of the two, heat or cold, cold therapy is believed to decrease pain faster and to have a longer-lasting effect than heat therapy. Contrast therapy, however, often works better than either one alone. It can be effective in reducing swelling, decreasing congestion, and improving organ function.

Therapeutic Massage for the Terminally Ill Patient

A gentle back rub can increase relaxation and ease the aches and pains associated with immobility. A slow, three-minute back rub can decrease heart rate and blood pressure, indicating relaxation. In one study, therapeutic massage was shown to be a beneficial nursing intervention that promotes relaxation and alleviates the perception of pain and anxiety in some cancer patients. A mild massage can increase superficial circulation to the area of treatment. As muscles are rubbed, blood return to the heart increases. Toxins such as lactic acid are removed from the muscle tissue and excreted from the body. Massage also has a sedative effect on the nervous system, reduces some types of swelling, and increases peristalsis (intestinal movement) thereby aiding digestion and decreasing constipation. When done correctly, therapeutic massage is said to trigger the release of endorphins in the brain that produce natural pain relievers by binding to opiate receptor sites involved in pain perception. *Although this action may increase one's threshold of pain, massage therapy should never be used as a substitute for the patient's routine analgesics.*

Massage therapy is contraindicated in areas where patients have varicose veins, blood clots, phlebitis (inflammation of the vein), open wounds, bruises, broken bones, cysts, or skin that was exposed to radiation therapy. Always consult the patient's physician or hospice nurse before beginning massage therapy. Some medical insurance companies partially pay for treatments by licensed massage therapists. Check with your patient's insurance company to see if this applies. Some licensed massage therapists have taken additional course work in order to better serve hospice patients. Inquire if there is one in your area.

A ten-minute gentle massage to the head, neck, limbs, and back can promote relaxation and a better night's sleep for your patient. Use a lubricant that is alcohol-free and does not absorb too quickly into the skin to avoid friction and skin irritation. Massage oils of various qualities can be purchased at health food stores or specialty shops, or you can combine a mixture of oils and scents just suitable to your patient's needs. Essential oils may be added to the base lubricant to include the benefits of aromatherapy along with the massage. Four parts unprocessed vegetable oil and one part almond oil and several drops of an appropriate essential oil can create a very soothing combination. Other oils that can be used as base oil include avocado, lanolin, safflower, and sunflower.

According to Srutakirti Das, who served as Srila Prabhupada's personal servant for several years, Srila Prabhupada liked his daily massage with mustard seed oil on his body and sandalwood oil on his head. Sometimes Srila Prabhupada requested that the mustard oil be mixed with camphor, and occasionally he requested the mustard oil be heated.

For added therapeutic effects, a teaspoon of the following oils can be added to the base oil as desired:

- Aloe Vera oil is known for its skin healing properties.

- Jojoba oil is known as an excellent skin moisturizer.

- Apricot kernel oil is also a very good skin moisturizer.

- Primrose oil is known for toning and adding vitamins.

After you have chosen and mixed your massage oil, transfer it into a plastic squeeze bottle. Fill a bowl with hot water and place the bottle of mixed lubricant in the water for about ten minutes so that, when applied, the lubricating oil is warm and soothing. Have a sheet or blanket on hand, because oils tend to lower body temperature. Remove any rings, bracelets, watches, etc. before beginning the massage so your patient's skin does not become scratched or irritated. Your hands should be clean and fingernails short.

Basic Techniques

Arrange for a quiet, peaceful setting in which to give a massage. The room should be warm, dimly lit, and very quiet. The patient may prefer silence or a soft chanting tape as background sound vibration. An aromatherapy candle may be lit for relaxation if oxygen therapy is not in use. Assist the patient into a comfortable position. If he is uncomfortable on his stomach, assist him in a side-lying position with knees bent. Extend one knee slightly so knees are not touching.

A good rule of thumb is that rapid, circular movements tend to stimulate the patient while smooth, slow strokes tend to promote relaxation. Move smoothly and rhythmically. Random movements with your hands will not feel very relaxing to the patient.

The Three-Minute Back Rub—Option 1

Use slow, rhythmic stroking on both sides of the backbone. To maintain continuous hand contact on your patient's skin, slowly and gently rub your left hand downward to the left of the spinal column. Before lifting your hand when it reaches the base of the back, begin a slow, rhythmic stroking with your right hand downward to the right of the spine moving slowly to the base of the back. Repeat this pattern for three minutes.

The Three-Minute Back Rub—Option 2

Use both thumbs to make a gentle, overlapping motion to massage the muscles in the upper back. Work on one side of the spine at a time. Maintain skin contact by pressing one thumb down just before lifting the other. For the last 30 seconds or so, use a slow, rhythmic stroke upward toward the shoulder blades.

The Three-Minute Back Rub—Option 3

With the patient on his stomach, stand at his waist. Reach across and place both of your palms on the side opposite you. Slowly and rhythmically, slide one palm, then the other, using a hand-over-hand motion. Constant skin contact is maintained by not lifting one hand before sliding the other hand. After a minute or so, move around to the other side of the bed and repeat this hand-over-hand motion for another minute or two.

The Ten-Minute Body Massage

Cover the patient with a bath towel draped across him or a folded sheet so that only the area being massaged is exposed. Position yourself at the head of the bed. With the patient lying on his back, gently cradle his head and neck in the palms of your hands. Help him to release any tension by gently turning his head to the right and then to the left. Bend it forward, and then back. Carefully place his head on a soft pillow. Use your fingertips, not your fingernails, to massage the scalp. Slowly rub bony prominences in the back of the head. Use your fingertips to massage both sides of the forehead. Stroke fingers across the forehead again and again until all signs of tension are gone. Move downward, gently stroking each eyebrow, the jaw, and chin.

Reposition yourself to the side of the bed. Use slow, rhythmic strokes while gently massaging the right arm, moving downward to his hand, fingers, in between each finger and finally each fingertip. Move to the other side of the bed. Repeat the same slow strokes going down the left arm to the hand, fingers, etc.

Position yourself next to the patient's right leg. Gently move your hands to his foot. Massage the top and bottom of the foot, massage each toe, and between the toes. Repeat this process on the left leg, foot, toes, etc.

Assist the patient to roll on his side so his back is exposed. Finish this body massage with a gentle, relaxing back rub.

In a hospice setting, therapeutic massage has been shown to enhance relaxation and comfort for some patients. It is a sensitive and caring exchange between the patient and caregiver. When teaching family members how to administer a basic back rub to a loved one, I have personally seen how this exchange can relieve caregivers of feelings of helplessness. This is a very personal way of serving and comforting the dying Vaishnava.

Srila Prabhupada's Remedies

When I joined the International Society for Krishna Consciousness (ISKCON) in 1972, an older godsister gave me a copy of natural remedies that Srila Prabhupada had shared with his disciples during the movement's earlier days. I have included the ones that may be relevant to hospice care, depending on the patient's symptoms and disease. Consult the patient's physician or hospice nurse before administering any of these treatments, as some ingredients may be contraindicated. (For example, ingestion of chili peppers or black pepper might be contraindicated in certain stomach or intestinal disorders.)

Common Cold

Srila Prabhupada's Cold Remedy #1: Add ½ teaspoon of crushed chili and a 1-inch piece of ginger root (diced) to 1½ cups of water. Bring to a boil. Add 1 teaspoon milk and 1 tablespoon honey. Allow chili to settle to the bottom before drinking. This loosens and clears nasal mucus associated with the common cold. The drink should be taken frequently during the day.

Srila Prabhupada's Cold Remedy #2: Combine 1 cup water and 1 teaspoon ground cloves. Gargle with mixture.

Srila Prabhupada's Cold Remedy #3: Peel a 1-inch piece of ginger root and cut into small pieces. Have the patient chew each piece, extracting the ginger root juice. (Chewed ginger root does not need to be swallowed.) Repeat four to five times a day.

Chest Cold and Congestion

Srila Prabhupada's Chest Cold Remedy #1: Fry ½ cup urad dal (a legume found in Indian grocery stores) in 2 tablespoons mustard seed oil. Allow mixture to cool to a warm but comfortable temperature. Apply warm mixture to chest, neck, hands, and bottom of feet before going to bed. In the morning, heat ½ cup water, 1 tablespoon honey, and ½ teaspoon ground ginger. Sip tea while still warm.

Srila Prabhupada's Chest Cold Remedy #2: Mix mustard seed oil and camphor. Apply to back, neck, chest, hands, and bottom of feet. Massage in well.

Srila Prabhupada's Chest Cold Remedy #3: Mix 1 tablespoon honey with ¼ teaspoon ground ginger. Eat frequently during the day.

Constipation
Drink a cup or two of hot milk. Prepare milk with honey or molasses instead of sugar as an added laxative.

Diarrhea
Drink ½ cup plain yogurt as tolerated.

Headache
For a simple headache, Srila Prabhupada suggested the following: Fill a teaspoon halfway with ground black pepper. Put a few drops of water on top of the pepper and mix gently. Heat the spoon by holding it directly over a flame on the stove until the mixture bubbles slightly and becomes a paste. If mixture is too thick, add a little more water. Cool until black pepper mixture can be comfortably touched. Apply mixture to the forehead.

Sore Muscles
Massage affected areas with a mixture of mustard seed oil and camphor.

Sore Throat
Combine 1 cup of water with 1 tablespoon ginger. Gargle frequently.

Stomach ache Caused by Indigestion
Chew a handful of anise seeds or roast a handful of cumin seeds and eat them when cooled.

Swollen Glands
Mix calcium carbonate with honey to a smooth thick paste. Do not make the mixture too watery. Apply to swollen glands at intervals during the day.

Toothache
Apply a few drops of oil of cloves to tooth and gum area to decrease pain while awaiting care from a dental professional.

This chapter has provided a brief explanation of some alternative and complementary therapies. The reader is encouraged to explore this subject matter in more depth if further detail is warranted. Although previously stated, due to its gravity, one point deserves mentioning again: *Because the patient's well-being is of prime importance, always consult with the primary physician and/or hospice nurse before beginning any additional therapies not already a part of his medical regimen.*

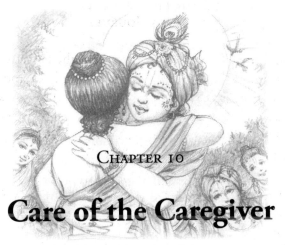

Chapter 10

Care of the Caregiver

*"You may not be able to do much to help your patients,"
a college professor once told me,
"but never leave them worse than you found them."*

Although his advice seemed somewhat flippant at the time, his words often haunted me at the end of a trying shift at the inpatient hospice unit. Had I relieved my patient's physical pain as well as I could have? Had I really stopped to listen to my patient's concerns and fears?

When I began home hospice care as a nurse, I found that visits were usually brief—yet it was not uncommon to stay, unexpectedly, at a patient's home for hours at a time. Often, family members required more emotional support than the patient. Some were angry at their sudden increase in responsibilities, and as a visiting nurse I sometimes took the brunt of their anger. Many times, it appeared that a family structure was so fragile it could fall apart at any moment, leaving the patient without any assistance. For those patients who were emotionally isolated from family, friends, and neighbors, as their nurse I became their only source of emotional support. A quick visit sometimes turned into an entire afternoon.

In addition, ministerial duties became part of my unwritten job description. One husband, a devout Catholic and the only caregiver for his terminally ill wife, confessed his guilt at having silently prayed for his wife's death to come swiftly, not only for her sake, but also because he was so tired. I had to reassure him that he was not the only caregiver to have ever felt this way. Still, the guilt tore him apart. His remorse at having prayed like this continued to torment him and after his wife's death he was inconsolable. I often drove away from my patients' homes taking these stressors with me.

Then I found myself on the opposite end of the fence. Unexpectedly, I became the primary caregiver for my own family member when my mother-in-law was diagnosed with inoperable cancer. My husband's eight brothers and sisters were counting on me to keep their mother out of pain. My mother-in-law would not allow the visiting hospice nurse to make a medical decision without first consulting me. Unlike the stressors I experienced as a hospice nurse, I now understood firsthand the physical and emotional exhaustion associated with caring for a loved one. I truly understood the turmoil and distress experienced by the families I had once tried to console.

Towards the end of my mother-in-law's life, I sat at her bedside for hours as she became more and more unresponsive to the world around her. I watched for the slightest sign of distress. A sudden increase in respirations or a soft moan were seen as communication of pain and were responded to quickly. I placed her rosary beads in her hand because I knew it would bring her spiritual comfort. I asked the priest from her church to visit and pray with her and for her. I sang soft *bhajans* to her as she lay still in her bed. But as she grew physically weaker, so did I. I was tired and emotionally exhausted. I remembered the elderly man who confessed his guilt at having prayed for his wife's death to come swiftly, not only for her sake, but also for his. I finally understood.

Having experienced both caregiver roles, one as a nurse and the other as a family member, I am very aware of the stressors that can contribute to caregiver burnout. The ordeal of the caregiver can be compared to a fire that starts out burning strong and bright but diminishes in size and strength if not given proper care. A caregiver's physical, emotional, mental, and spiritual stamina can become tested in so many ways that over time, his or her brilliance and strength can be reduced to what seems like nothing more than ashes.

Much research has been done on internal and external stressors experienced by hospice professionals and others in the caring profession. In an article written by Dale G. Larson, Ph.D., from the University of Santa Clara in California, "helper secrets" were gathered from 200 hospice workers and analyzed to better understand the stressors involved in working with those whose death was imminent. I have included a few "helper secrets" revealed by hospice professionals, because some of these thoughts emanating from sheer mental and physical exhaustion are universal, meaning that they can be experienced not only by those working in the hospice field, but also by those caregivers who put their personal lives on hold, so to speak, while caring for a dying loved one.

Some "helper secrets" revealed were as follows:

- "I may be too selfish to do this work."

- "Sometimes I ignore the needs of my patient because I know I can't fulfill them completely."

- "I think of humorous, sarcastic answers to my patient's painful questions or comments."

- "I have distanced myself deliberately from my patient and his family as a form of self-protection when I have felt emotionally overloaded, even though I felt they needed emotional support."

- "Sometimes I pray that God takes this patient because he is suffering so much. I hope he dies soon. I feel guilty."

Caregivers are natural helpers. We are more than willing to assist others and feel good about helping those around us. But to assist one who is dying is a tremendous undertaking. Problems often arise when the expectations we place upon ourselves become unrealistic and humanly impossible. What we expect of ourselves and what we wish for our patients may simply be unattainable. There is often a wide gap between how we envision ourselves as caregivers and the grueling tasks we must attend to every day. We can comfort others just so much. We can sit at someone's bedside for just so long. We can deprive ourselves of rest for just so many hours. At some point, hopefully sooner than later, we must realize that without giving ourselves "care" we will be of no use to the people we are trying to help.

According to Larson, when a caregiver's self-expectations are not met, it often results in guilt, anxiety, resentment, and anger. The result is burnout, which is experienced by the caregiver when he or she is unable to successfully adapt to and cope with perceived stressors.

Stressors can be exogenous (external) or endogenous (internal). An example of an exogenous stressor in a caregiver situation might include loud traffic noise that is keeping your patient awake at night. An example of an endogenous stressor in a caregiver situation might include you, the caregiver, envisioning yourself as anticipating your patient's every need before he has to ask for it. Obviously, this would be impossible, but if you expected this of yourself, it might become an endogenous stressor. Whether originating internally or externally, an anxiety reaction to these stressors depends on the caregiver's perception of these experiences. Over time, the extent to which stress is perceived or experienced may affect one physically, mentally, emotionally, and spiritually.

On the subject of burnout prevention, Porter Storey, MD, a hospice physician, has identified warning signs of caregiver burnout. Reaction to stress will vary with each individual, but some common warning signs to look for are as follows:

- Weight loss or gain
- Frequent headaches
- Gastrointestinal disturbances
- Muscle tightness or strain
- Inability to sleep
- Anger
- Irritability
- Frustration
- Depression
- Guilt
- Feelings of overwhelming responsibility
- Feelings of helplessness and an inability to cope
- Feelings of inadequacy or insecurity

Avoiding Caregiver Burnout

Although it is difficult, it is essential to identify early warning signs of caregiver stress and to intervene before it becomes burnout. Just as one's reaction to stressors will vary, ways of managing our stress will vary as well. Some recommendations include:

- Maintain regular, healthy meals.

- Arrange for caregiver relief so adequate sleep is maintained. If you are not able to arrange for regular nighttime coverage, it is recommended that a regulated sleep pattern be maintained as much as possible. This will often present a challenge. If you are only able to arrange caregiver relief during the day, then try to rest at that same time every day.

- Take a break. This may include asking another caregiver to replace you, even for a few minutes, or take a short break while your patient is asleep. Find a few moments to be alone each day.

- Chant *japa* while taking a break or while sitting at your patient's bedside. Surely, maintaining your *sadhana* that was upheld prior to your caregiver responsibilities will be difficult. However, tremendous spiritual stamina will be gained by continuing to chant your prescribed number of rounds of *japa*. Whenever possible, find a few minutes to sing *bhajans* or read a verse and purport from Srila Prabhupada's transcendental books. Spend a few quiet moments praying to the Lord.

- Remind yourself that Lord Krishna is the source of all strength, both physically and spiritually. In the *Bhagavad-gita*, the Lord states, "I am the strength of the strong." (BG 10.36) Write this quotation on a large piece of paper and mount it where you can see it often during the day.

- Forgive yourself for committing mistakes. The terminally ill do not expect us to be infallible. They only ask that we do not abandon them.

- Reveal your mind in confidence to someone you trust. This is one of the six loving exchanges between Vaishnavas. It is not a sign of weakness to ask for help, but a sign of great strength.

- Define realistic expectations of yourself.

- If it is helpful, keep a personal journal of your thoughts and realizations while caring for your patient. This is also a way to preserve the memory of the dying Vaishnava you are caring for and may comfort you after her death. In caring for a loved one, we become forced, often painfully, to find meaning in a most difficult situation. Keeping a journal may help with your search.

As a caregiver, it is essential to find what it is that gives you the inner strength to hold up another person. As a useful metaphor, imagine that you, the caregiver, are hanging on the edge of a cliff with one hand and trying to lift up your patient with the other. Certainly you would never think of letting go of the cliff or you would both fall. Finding a way to hold on to your source of strength while lifting up your patient is the key to avoiding caregiver burnout.

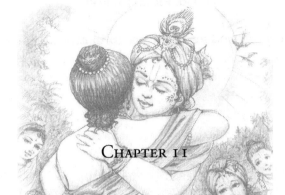

Chapter 11

Signs and Symptoms of Approaching Death

When a man is dying, the walls of his room enclose a chapel, and it is right to enter it in hushed reverence.
—Sherwin B. Nuland in **How We Die**

The difference between a sign and a symptom is that one is usually thought to be objective and the other subjective. In general, a sign is objective evidence of a disease or disorder that can be seen, heard, felt, or measured. A symptom is generally thought to be subjective and includes information from the patient such as the onset of pain, precipitating causes, location, severity, and relieving factors.

Just as there are signs and symptoms of a disease, there are many signs and symptoms of approaching death in a terminally ill patient. Although the dying process is as unique as the individual experiencing it, I have seen many of these signs manifest in a similar way despite the original cause of illness. The time line for these signs and symptoms is a flexible one with changes generally beginning anywhere from one to three months before death occurs.

Two separate but interdependent processes will often take place. One is on a physical level, in which the body's systems slowly shut down, and the other is on a mental, emotional, and spiritual level, in which the patient distances herself from the world around her. Usually within a month or two before death, many patients shift from intellectualizing about their terminal condition to a true comprehension and acceptance of their mortality.

Decreased socialization often occurs at this time, so patients may become more quiet and withdrawn. Your patient may be trying to detach himself from his surroundings and those around him in order to "let go." This progression of behavior is not exclusive to Vaishnavas and seems to occur in many patients no matter what spiritual or religious affiliation they adhere to. Your patient may indicate a desire to be alone more often or ask to see only a few people. Reassure family and friends that being one of the people he requests to see is, quite often, an indication of who he needs support from at this particular time and not necessarily a sign of who he loves or appreciates the most. It may also be someone the patient needs to see in order to reach an emotional closure.

A terminally ill patient who is feeling more withdrawn may not feel the need to verbalize her realizations and reasons for solitude. If this is the case, her silence can sometimes create, unintentionally, new dynamics within the family. Loved ones often perceive the patient as "pushing them away." This can lead to anger and resentment on the part of the family, who may feel rejected after having given so much of themselves to the patient's care. As a caregiver, you may be able to lessen existing tension by gently reminding loved ones that the patient's withdrawal is a natural and necessary part of the dying process. It is not that the patient is ungrateful for the help she has received, but that she needs to separate herself from those around her in order to complete her journey. This is an internal passage in which the patient must travel alone.

In addition, periods of **rest and sleep increase** for the patient at this time. Even while awake, he may lay for hours in silence with his eyes closed. Encourage those involved to respect the patient's need for quiet and seclusion. Reassure them that nonverbal communication through a gentle touch on the hand can speak volumes.

Further Signs of Approaching Death

When family and friends are aware of the bodily and mental changes that may occur in a terminally ill patient, it sometimes alleviates the fears that come from seeing a loved one in this condition. Some of the signs listed below may or may not appear in all patients, may appear in a different order, and will certainly not appear all at once. If present, they will become more apparent and worsen during the final few days of life.

Sometimes within weeks or even months of death, it is not uncommon for the terminally ill patient to **speak to someone who has already died or to those you cannot see**. Often this can be attributed to lack of oxygen to the brain, a disease process such as brain cancer or metastasis, or a medication reaction. It is difficult, however, to understand the detachment process that occurs at the end of one's life, and hospice professionals often see these events as a sign that death is imminent. While working in the inpatient hospice unit, we nurses passed on these patient experiences to the oncoming staff as routinely as the patient's vital signs. We never argued with the patients about what they claimed to see or hear. Unless we could medically prove otherwise, we simply viewed these events as another step closer in their transition.

This "awareness" that often occurs when someone is close to death may involve a patient indicating when her death will take place. These verbal "clues" are often missed by family and friends but remembered later on after the patient has passed away. For example, I cared for a man who stated in the summer, "The holidays will be an unhappy time at my house this year." He passed away two days before Christmas.

In this regard, it should be noted that some patients who are nearing death appear to wait until a significant date before passing away, such as the birth of a grandchild or a milestone birthday. A woman dying of cancer would often speak to me about her upcoming birthday. Considering the extent of her disease, it seemed impossible that she could live long enough to reach that date. She passed away the evening of her ninetieth birthday with her family at her bedside.

Another common theme seen by those who care for the terminally ill is that patients sometimes wait for the presence of a particular person before passing away, or they may wait for someone to not be present. For example, I stayed by my mother-in-law's bedside the entire night before she passed away. Her youngest daughter, whom she always protected, was there as well. My sister-in-law stayed through most of the night, often sleeping with her head on her mother's lap. I sensed it would be extremely difficult for such a loving mother to die in the presence of the daughter she had sheltered for so long. I finally suggested that my sister-in-law rest for a while in another room. Shortly after, as the sun began to rise, my mother-in-law passed away. This phenomenon seems to occur quite often. Many families have reported stepping out of the room for "just a few minutes," only to return and find their loved one had passed away in that very short amount of time.

One young devotee dying of cancer had asked her sister to chant Hare Krishna at the time of her death if she was unable to do so herself. Without the association of other Vaishnavas, her last days were spent in the hospital, nonverbal and unresponsive. Her parents and sister stayed with her day and night. Eventually, when her parents stepped out of the room for only a few moments, her sister remembered what she was previously asked to do and began to chant the Hare Krishna mantra. Within minutes, this fortunate soul squeezed her sister's hand and passed away peacefully while hearing the Lord's holy names.

As the time of death approaches, your patient may exhibit increased **restlessness and/or repetitive actions**, such as pulling at bed linens or repeatedly reaching for something in the air that is not visible to anyone else but the patient. This is sometimes referred to as "terminal anxiety." You may also observe **increased confusion** as time passes. For the devotee, hearing the chanting of the Hare Krishna mantra or listening to a soft *bhajan* recording may decrease the restlessness often experienced in this later stage of a terminal disease. Reading Krishna's pastimes aloud may also help to ease anxiety. Speak calmly and assuredly and never in a tone which can be taken by the patient as condescending. Soft lighting and decreased environmental noise and other stimuli may help to relax your patient as well.

Decreased Eating and Drinking

As the sense of taste changes, patients will naturally lose interest in eating. Eating and drinking will also decrease as digestion slows and swallowing becomes more difficult. During his final days, when he is no longer able to eat but can still tolerate liquids, keep your patient's mouth moist with sips of cool water through a straw, or give small pieces of ice chips with a teaspoon. This will be a comfort to your patient as long as he can tolerate it without coughing or choking. Be sure the head of the bed is elevated or that the patient's head and chest are lifted with pillows before administering even the smallest amount of liquid or ice chips. Lips should be kept moist by applying a nonpetroleum-based lubricant, such as K-Y Jelly, every few hours. If oxygen is not being administered, then Vaseline can be applied. Moisten lips and the inside of the mouth every two hours with cool water by using a disposable, sponge-like "toothette." During the last few days of life when even small sips can cause choking, he will most likely have no fluid intake. This is most difficult for family members to accept. It should be explained to them, however, that natural dehydration is a part of the dying process and is not painful for the patient. Never force foods or fluids, as this will not make your patient comfortable at this time. The body is now conserving energy for more important needs.

Incontinence

If your patient was previously continent of bowel and bladder, she may experience loss of control of this function as her disease progresses. Whether or not an indwelling catheter is in place, urine output will gradually decrease. It may darken in color, contain blood, or thicken in consistency as fluid intake decreases and kidney function begins to cease. Keeping the skin clean and dry and applying a thick, protective moisture barrier cream will prevent rashes and other skin breakdown that can result from incontinence. Disposable or washable briefs for adults are sometimes necessary to achieve this result. As always, be sensitive to any care that may cause indignities for your patient. Placing a thick padded cloth under the patient and changing it regularly may assist in keeping her just as clean. Even a patient who has stopped eating and drinking may have some output of urine or bowel. In the last few days of life, however, it is not uncommon for a patient to have very little or no output at all. Most likely, the hospice nurse or other medical professional will palpate the patient's lower abdomen to see if the bladder is distended. This will indicate whether or not she is retaining urine or has simply slowed down her output.

Vital Signs and Skin Color begin to Change

As the body's systems begin to shut down, the patient's **blood pressure** may decrease. **Pulse** rate will often increase (normal pulse is about 70 beats per minute), or it may decrease to well below 60 beats per minute. Radial pulses (felt in the wrists) may feel weak and be difficult to locate. Pedal pulses (felt on the feet) may be undetectable. The patient's **skin** may become moist and clammy. As the caregiver, continue to keep the patient clean and dry. A tepid bed bath will be quite refreshing to your patient at this time. Be sure the bed linens are changed often if the patient is perspiring. If the back of his head and neck become moist with perspiration, place a small towel on his pillow to absorb excess moisture. Unless he feels cold, apply a cool washcloth to his forehead. Dab his face with the cloth from time to time. The washcloth will become warm quickly, so rinse it with cool water at least every hour or two. Body **temperature** may fluctuate between a high fever and below normal temperatures. Normal body temperature average is 36.2 degrees Celsius (98.6 degrees Fahrenheit), and is usually maintained between 35.6 degrees Celsius to 37.8 degrees Celsius (96 degrees - 100 degrees Fahrenheit). The patient's arms, hands and legs may become cool to touch. As death nears, you may notice a **mottling** in skin color on the patient's heels, knees, or ears. Mottling appears like small areas of purplish discoloration and is caused by decreased circulation. It may continue down the patient's legs or be seen on other parts of the body as well. The underside of the body may become darker in color and nail beds often become bluish. These are other signs of blood circulation slowing down.

Change in Breathing Pattern

Toward the end of life, your patient's respirations will most likely change. Her lungs may begin to fill with fluid and her breathing may sound moist. Normally, a person breathes 16-20 times per minute. At the end stage, respirations can be shallow and can increase to over 40 breaths per minute. You may notice apnea, periods without breathing, which can last for as little as ten seconds or as long as one minute or two. The apnea will then cease and respirations will resume as before. Your patient may "mouth breathe," inhaling and exhaling through the mouth rather than the nose, or she may exhale as if blowing air through closed lips. For comfort and to increase lung capacity, keep the head of the bed elevated or elevate her head and chest with pillows. Turning the patient slightly on her side with her head and chest elevated may help her to breathe with less effort. Fold a pillow in half lengthwise and gently wedge it behind her to assist with positioning. Reposition her at least every two hours for comfort and to avoid pressure sores. If the patient's breathing becomes more of an endeavor while lying on her side, immediately reposition her on her back.

As always, the head and chest should be elevated at least 45-60 degrees, or higher if needed. If oxygen is being administered, be sure the nasal prongs are in place. If a small electric fan is available, place it on a low speed and direct it towards your patient's face from a comfortable distance. Be sure the patient has adequate, natural circulation of air in the room.

A Few Days to Hours before Death

Eventually your patient may become nonverbal and may not respond to external stimuli, such as talking or light touch. **Not every hospice patient enters this stage, but most patients I have cared for have.** Some hospice professionals refer to this end stage as "actively dying." The patient may appear to be in a coma-like state but has most likely entered this final stage of the dying process. The longest I have seen a patient remain in this stage was six days, but that was very unusual. Typically, patients will remain in an "actively dying" stage from 24 to 72 hours. Even though he may not respond, your patient can still hear you and others. Be sure nothing is said in his presence that you would not want him to hear. **For a devotee, continuous chanting of the Hare Krishna mantra should be performed at this crucial time.**

Srila Prabhupada writes, "If one somehow or other remembers the holy name of Narayana, Krishna, or Rama at the end of life, he immediately achieves the transcendental result of going back home, back to Godhead." (SB 8.1.48)

Whether or not your patient is unresponsive to verbal or other stimuli, pain medications for comfort should be continued. By now, pain and other necessary medications that were previously administered orally should have been converted to more tolerable routes such as sublingual or transdermal. Even though your patient cannot verbalize her pain, it does not mean she is not feeling discomfort. Continue administering pain medicine and other medications for comfort as prescribed by the physician.

The following signs of impending death may or may not occur, but if present, are indications that the patient will probably pass away within a day or two or even within hours:

- The patient's breathing may become slower. His lungs may fill with fluid, making each breath sound as though he is under water. This "rattling sound" is caused by accumulation of secretions in the large airways and is sometimes referred to as the "death rattle." Because the patient is too weak to cough, secretions may also collect in the back of his throat and airway. These secretions are normal and consist of saliva, mucous, and any other liquids that are introduced into the patient's mouth, such as water from toothettes or liquid medication.

- Normally, a healthy person is able to clear the throat and swallow or spit any excess secretions. At the end of life, however, a person may become too weak to clear his throat and swallow secretions. Altered levels of consciousness, such as when a patient is lethargic or comatose, may also impair a patient's ability to clear his airway, causing secretions to build up. This causes a rattling sound when air passes through the airway. This sound may get louder as each hour passes.

- While there is no definitive way of knowing how these secretions affect a patient's comfort when he is actively dying and unable to speak, we can only hope that the discomfort is minimal. The increasingly louder sounds he makes may become extremely disturbing to loved ones.

What can you Do?

There are a few practical things you can do to help minimize or even eliminate the "death rattle."

Reposition your patient. Sometimes turning a person from her back to her side will be enough to clear excess secretions from the airway. In addition, raise the head of the bed to help promote drainage.

Decrease the amount of water intake. Keep your patient's lips, as well as the inside of his mouth, moist with wet sponges (toothettes). However, minimize the amount of water that will drain down the throat by squeezing excess water from the sponge before using it.

Give anti-cholinergic medicine as prescribed by the physician. Anti-cholinergic medications, such as atropine or scopolamine, help dry up excess secretions, thus decreasing the loud rattling sound when breathing.

- Apnea may be present more often and for longer periods of time. This chaotic pattern of breathing, consisting of periods of apnea followed by increased depth and frequency of respiration, is called Cheyne-Stokes respiration.

- The patient's skin may feel cooler to the touch and may appear bluish in her hands and feet. Mottling may increase at this stage and may be seen in the knees, ankles, or elbows. Discoloration can travel down the legs or other parts of the body within hours and is a sign of further decrease in circulation.

- The patient's eyes may remain open or partially open and may have a fixed stare without blink reflex. The pupils may have a glassy appearance. An occasional tear may flow from the tear ducts but is not necessarily an indication of the patient crying.

- Although it is recommended that we do not bother a patient at this time by taking vital signs, it may be necessary to know that, during this final stage, his blood pressure will probably decrease and his pulses may feel weaker and more difficult to locate. Body temperature is usually below normal, but I have had patients whose temperatures rose to 105 degrees Fahrenheit the night before they passed away.

Assisting your Patient with Closure

Even when patients are in the "actively dying" stage, some may linger for days, enduring severe physical stressors, as if waiting for something to be said or someone to arrive.

I recall a 28-year-old gentleman dying of an AIDS-related illness. For several days he remained nonverbal and struggled for each breath. Finally, his father, a devout minister who had disapproved of his son's lifestyle, came to his bedside. Sensing that this was the person my patient was probably waiting to see, I told his father, "He has been waiting for you, sir. Please tell him everything you need to tell him, and if you are able, tell him what he needs to hear. Please give him permission to 'let go.'"

With tears in his eyes, his father softly whispered, "I am sorry for any pain I have caused you, son. I always loved you. Now it's time for you to go in peace."

My patient took his last breath and passed away.

Like this young man, I have seen many patients linger in the final stages of life until loved ones told them something they needed to hear. Sensitivity to these matters of closure for a dying person is essential in hospice care. For a devotee, this principle also applies.

Life's unfinished business can take many forms, and anxiety over unresolved issues may manifest in various ways. We each have within us a storehouse filled with emotional truths that are based on our conditioning and personal experiences. During the time you cared for your patient, she may or may not have required your assistance in dealing with such matters. She may have been more comfortable reaching her own conclusions. Perhaps she was unaware of what issues needed to be resolved in her life or was unwilling or unable to discuss them.

Whatever the situation, if your patient seems to be lingering in the "actively dying" stage, it is not unusual for caregivers and other loved ones to feel frustrated, with a deep sense of helplessness. As an intimate caregiver, however, you may have gotten to know your patient so well that, to your own amazement, you can successfully anticipate what he requires for emotional closure before death, as described above with my young patient and his father. Of course, it is not always possible to understand what our patients require in this regard. Recalling past conversations with your patient may help you understand what he needs to finalize before successfully leaving this world. The emotional and psychological needs of the Vaishnava patient must never be minimized or ignored. Our goal in caring for the dying devotee is to provide holistic comfort in his final days so he can concentrate his mind on the Lord. To have come this far in caring for the terminally ill devotee and then to intentionally or unintentionally diminish his emotional needs would be a tremendous disservice.

If your patient is married, with children, and especially young children, she may benefit from having her family reassure her that they will be able to carry on once she is gone. Often this provides a patient with the peace of mind she needs to concentrate on more spiritual matters. If agreeable, allow each family member a few minutes of privacy with the patient. If you, the caregiver, are a family member, afford yourself this opportunity as well. Even though a patient may be nonverbal and unresponsive, she can still be reassured about any final anxieties that may be holding her back from an undisturbed and spiritual departure from this world.

As previously stated, not all patients enter this "actively dying" stage. In December 2000, in the holy land of Vrindavan, India, our society of devotees, as well as the world in general, lost a very dear Vaishnava named Ram Das. Ram Das Prabhu was a kind and enthusiastic devotee who served as head *pujari* for fourteen years in the ISKCON Los Angeles temple. He was loved and respected by all who knew him and will always be remembered for his gentle and compassionate ways.

After being diagnosed with a terminal heart condition, Ram Das moved to Vrindavan to live out his final days with his wife, Krsna Kumari Dasi. In a letter I received dated March 23, 2001, she wrote:

> On his last day, Ram Das Prabhu read scripture most of the day. In the evening he had two guests, Kavichandra Swami and Bali Dasa. They chatted about all kinds of philosophical concepts while (Kavichandra) Maharaja performed reiki on Ram Das for three hours. The guests left at 9 p.m., and Ram Das had his milk and pills. I called the doctor to inform him of Ram's condition, because at that point he was monitoring him daily. When I walked back into the room where Ram was sitting, he said, 'I'll be all right. You just go to bed.'
>
> I could see that the process was already starting, so I sat beside him and helped him hold his favorite picture of Srila Prabhupada's feet on his chest. I told him, 'Everything is all right. Srila Prabhupada is here,' which was true in every sense, as just fifteen minutes before a friend had returned to us a very large photo of Srila Prabhupada. I had joked at the door, 'Oh look, Srila Prabhupada is here!'
>
> Fluid was quickly filling Ram's lungs and I called out, 'Say Krishna! Chant!' He began to chant, although it was actually humanly impossible. He turned his face and looked at Srila Prabhupada and said, 'Krishna!' and then left very peacefully... He taught me how to be grateful to everyone and to give everyone I see a smile and 'Hari bol.' Of course, he is famous for his 'Remember, Krishna loves you.'... He gave of himself tirelessly to any and all, at all hours of the day and night. He was very rare.

We can learn from this example how important it is for the primary caregiver to maintain a calm and spiritual atmosphere during the last few hours and moments of a person's life. Constantly hearing the chanting of the Hare Krishna mantra at the time of death is the "spiritual prescription" given to us by Srila Prabhupada and Lord Chaitanya Mahaprabhu.

Lord Krishna tells Arjuna, "And whoever, at the time of death, quits his body, remembering Me alone, at once attains My nature. Of this there is no doubt." (BG 8.5)

In his purport regarding this verse, Srila Prabhupada writes, "Anyone who quits his body in Krishna consciousness is at once transferred to the transcendental abode of the Supreme Lord... To remember Krishna one should chant the *maha mantra*, Hare Krishna, Hare Krishna, Krishna Krishna, Hare Hare, Hare Rama, Hare Rama, Rama Rama, Hare Hare, incessantly, following in the footsteps of Lord Chaitanya... In such a way one will be able to depart from the body successfully remembering Krishna and so attain the supreme goal."

If your patient is unable to chant the Hare Krishna mantra due to his advanced disease, it is the duty of the caregiver to continuously chant to him. This may have to be very close to the patient's ear if he is experiencing any type of hearing loss due to a disease process. A recording of Srila Prabhupada chanting *japa* can be played round the clock to ensure that the chanting remains constant. In this way, he will have the opportunity to hear the holy names of the Lord, meditate on His beautiful form, and remember His transcendental pastimes.

In the *Srimad-Bhagavatam* 5.3.12, Srila Prabhupada translates, "Dear Lord, we may not be able to remember Your name, form, and qualities due to stumbling, hunger, falling down, yawning, or being in a miserable diseased condition at the time of death when there is a high fever. We therefore pray unto You, O Lord, for You are very affectionate to Your devotees. Please help us remember You, and to utter Your holy names, attributes, and activities, which can dispel all the reactions of our sinful lives."

In his purport, Srila Prabhupada explains, "The real success in life is *ante narayana-smrti*—remembering the holy name, attributes, activities, and forms of the Lord at the time of death. Although we may be engaged in the Lord's devotional service in the temple, material conditions are so tough and inevitable that we may forget the Lord at the time of death due to a diseased condition or mental derangement. Therefore, we should pray to the Lord to be able to remember His lotus feet without fail at the time of death, when we are in such a precarious condition."

With each passing year, increasing numbers of devotees are leaving this world after battling with painful long-term illnesses. Some were actively engaged in devotional service before they passed away; others had traveled far from their service and distanced themselves from the community of devotees. In the end, however, many of these dying Vaishnavas returned to the welcoming and loving arms of their godbrothers and godsisters in order to spend their final days in the association of devotees. Although some became too ill to chant Hare Krishna themselves, these devotees received the Lord's mercy just the same. At the time of death, kindhearted Vaishnavas surrounded these dying devotees and chanted the holy name of the Lord to them as they peacefully passed away.

This mood of accommodating all devotees at the end of their lives was the inspiration for forming Vaisnavas C.A.R.E., Inc. (Counseling, Assistance, Resource, and Education for the Terminally Ill and their Families), a worldwide network of volunteers who offer emotional and spiritual assistance to terminally ill devotees in their communities by visiting the patients and families. Additionally, the group provides many other opportunities to offer services even from within one's own home; for example, prayer partners send in a weekly prayer for those in need of loving care and inspiration. For additional information about this project, please visit www.vaisnavascare.org.

His Holiness Indradyumna Swami writes in his book, *Diary of a Traveling Preacher* (Volume 3, Chapter 30), "It is important how one actually leaves this world. In one sense, a devotee's whole life is in preparation for that one moment. The consciousness at death determines one's next destination. There is a Bengali proverb: *Bhajan kara sadhana kara—murte janle hoy*: 'Whatever *bhajan* and *sadhana* one has performed throughout his life will be tested at the moment of death.' But what happens if a devotee cannot fix his mind on Krishna at the moment of death? A doctor recently told me that eighty percent of people are actually unconscious at the moment of death! The body 'naturally' goes into a state of shock before the traumatic moment when the soul leaves the body... Once Ramanujacarya, after the death of Yamunacarya, was pensive with some questions. He requested Kancipuma, the servant of Lord Varadaraja

(Krishna), to ask the Lord some questions on his behalf. One of the questions was, 'What happens if a devotee dies suddenly and is unable to think of You at the time of death?' Lord Varadaraja replied, 'Then I will think of My devotee.'"

How do you Know when Death has Occurred?

Respirations cease. Sometimes a patient will take what appears to be his last breath, with a final exhalation a few moments later.

- Heartbeat ceases.

- Pupils are fixed and dilated.

- Jaw may relax and mouth may remain slightly open.

- Eyelids may remain open.

Take note of the time of death. If a hospice nurse has overseen the patient's care, notify the hospice at this time. Country and state laws vary, but the nurse may be required to make a visit to pronounce the patient's death. Remain composed and support others who are present. Take solace in the fact that you have done an extraordinary service in caring for the dying devotee. You comforted her physically, emotionally, mentally, and spiritually throughout the last months of her life. And during her final moments, you assisted her with her journey back home, back to Krishna.

"The presence of a devotee at the time of death elevates even the killer of a *brahmana* to the spiritual sky." (*Hari Bhakti Vilasa* 10.86)

In a *Srimad-Bhagavatam* class given in Los Angeles in the early 1970s, I personally heard Srila Prabhupada describe, "For a devotee, death is just like sleeping. He closes his eyes and when he opens them, there is Krishna. It is so nice."

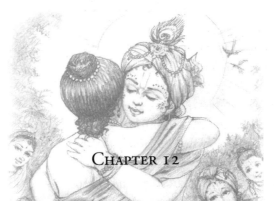

CHAPTER 12

Post-Mortem Care, Cremation Ceremony, and Memorial Service

Post-Mortem Care of the Vaishnava

As stated in the *Srimad-Bhagavatam,* our Vaishnava tradition recommends cremation of the body after death rather than burial. It is customary to cleanse and prepare the body in an auspicious manner for the cremation ceremony. Obviously, this would not be an easy task for a close family member or someone who is extremely distraught at this time. However, performing this sacred ritual can be beneficial in several ways, including assisting someone with emotional closure. Whoever performs this duty, however, should be very comfortable doing so. The Hare Krishna *maha-mantra* should be softly chanted throughout the ritual of preparing the body for cremation.

When a devotee has passed away, it is recommended to bathe the body with pure water from one of the sacred rivers of India, such as the Yamuna or Ganges. A small bottle of Ganges water can be purchased online from websites such as www.krishnaculture.com and www.amazon.com. Begin by pouring a small amount of holy water into a clean bowl or basin. Using a wash cloth, lightly wipe the body with the holy water. Pat dry with a towel. *Tilaka* should be applied to the 12 appropriate places on the body, while chanting the following mantras:

Nose and forehead: **om keshavaya namaha**
Abdomen: **om narayanaya namaha**
Chest: **om madhavaya namaha**

Throat: **om govindaya namaha**
Right Side: **om vishnave namaha**
Right Arm: **om madhusudanaya namah**a
Right Shoulder: **om trivikramaya namaha**
Left Side: **om vamanaya namaha**
Left Arm: **om shridharaya namah**a
Left Shoulder: **om hrshikeshaya namaha**
Upper Back: **om padmanabhaya namaha**
Lower Back: **om damodaraya namaha**

If possible, obtain sandalwood paste that has first been offered to the Deities and write the name of Krishna across the chest of the deceased. The devotee should then be dressed in new devotional clothes. Three things should now be placed in the mouth of the deceased: a *tulasi* leaf that has first been offered to the Lord, a few drops of *caranamrita* (bath water) from the Deities, and dust from the holy *dhama* of Vrindavan. Place a garland from the Deities around the neck. A small piece of clothing from the Deities is often pinned or tied to the upper portion of the devotee's clothes. A *harinama chaddar* can be wrapped around the upper body. The body can then be sprinkled with more holy water. This entire purification process before cremation is done with the feeling that we are surrendering the dead body into a sacred fire.

Cremation Ceremony in the West

The cremation ceremony should be performed at a crematorium where Vaishnava beliefs will be respected. Be aware that not all crematoriums will allow family members to be present when the body is placed in the cremation chamber. Be sure to ask before selecting a crematorium. Arrangements should be made ahead of time so that the body is cremated as soon as possible after the soul has departed. However, laws vary from state to state and country to country regarding how soon the cremation can take place after death. Your hospice staff should be knowledgeable about local regulations. If arrangements can be made for even a few family members and close friends to be present during the cremation, then chanting the Hare Krishna *maha-mantra* will bestow the greatest spiritual benefit upon the departed soul as well as everyone in attendance.

Memorial Service for the Vaishnava

Several years ago after a devotee passed away in an automobile accident, Srila Prabhupada wrote a letter to Revatinandana Das concerning a memorial service. An excerpt from this letter, dated November 14, 1973, follows:

> Regarding the auto accident, just hold a condolence meeting for Raghava Das Brahmacari and pray for his soul to Krishna for giving him a good chance for advancement in Krishna consciousness. Certainly Krishna will give him a good place to take birth where he can again begin in Krishna conscious activities. That is sure. But, we offer our condolences to a departed soul separated from a Vaishnava. Do you know that there must be *prasadam* distributed? Three days after the demise of a Vaishnava a function should be held for offering the departed soul and all others *prasada*. This is the system.

Srila Prabhupada again instructed the devotees on this matter after a devotee passed away in France. His Divine Grace advised the devotees to perform a *kirtan* at the memorial service, followed by a lecture from the *Bhagavad-gita* regarding the eternal nature of the soul. Anyone present may speak about the qualities of the departed Vaishnava, as well as his devotional activities and any other fond memories they may wish to share. At the conclusion of the service, a *prasadam* feast should be distributed in honor of the beloved Vaishnava. *(From a lecture given by His Holiness Indradyumna Swami in honor of a departed Vaishnava on 3/30/2001, Philadelphia)*

When they are able, many devotees from the West bring the ashes of the deceased to the holy *dhama* or they make an arrangement for someone else to bring the ashes. It is recommended that the ashes of the deceased be immersed in a holy river such as the Yamuna or Ganges within one year. According to Vaishnava tradition, this final act of care is a most auspicious spiritual service to the departed soul.

Remembering the Vaishnava

From reading the *Bhagavad-gita* we can understand that the Lord personally protects a soul who has taken shelter at His lotus feet, and at the time of death the Lord will never abandon His devotee. To remember and honor a departed loved one, family and friends can perform devotional service on the anniversary of his passing away. A service can be performed in memory of that departed soul that can include *arati* to the Deities, *kirtan*, and a *prasadam* feast distributed on his behalf. Here are some other suggestions:

- Offer a donation of money, cloth, jewelry, etc., to the Deities on behalf of the deceased.

- Sponsor a *puja*, flower garlands, or a new outfit for the Deities on behalf of the departed soul.

- Support a Sunday feast program or festival at one of Srila Prabhupada's temples in the name of your loved one.

- Plant a fruit or flowering tree in honor of the deceased and, when available, offer its fruits and flowers to the Deities.

- Gather with family and friends to hear *Bhagavad-gita*, share memories, and honor *prasadam* in loving tribute to the departed soul.

Whatever you choose to do to honor the departed Vaishnava on the anniversary of her passing away from this world, it is always recommended that the chanting of the Hare Krishna *maha-mantra* and *prasadam* distribution accompany your offering.

In this regard, when speaking about the passing away of Haridas Thakur, Srila Prabhupada stated in a lecture, "That means his funeral ceremony was conducted by Chaitanya Mahaprabhu Himself. He took the body to the seaside and in the graveyard He [conducted the funeral ceremony]...with *kirtan*. *Kirtan* is always there. And after burial there was distribution of *prasadam* and *kirtan*." (Lecture on April 5, 1967, San Francisco)

Please consult the appendices at the back of this book for detailed information about how to perform ash immersion ceremonies in Vrindavan and Mayapur, India, as well as more information about the traditional *sraddha* ceremony (memorial service).

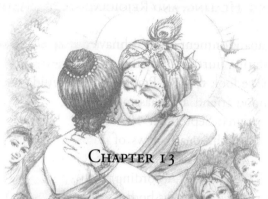

CHAPTER 13

Grieving, Healing, and Rejoicing for the Vaishnava

*"Whenever a devotee passes away,
this world becomes a little more unfortunate."*

—*Indradyumna Swami*

Caring for a friend or family member can be exhausting work that, unfortunately, does not abruptly end with the death of that loved one. Those who are left behind must endure and work through their grief in order to successfully emerge from such a deep loss. Reaching a healthy resolution, either for oneself or assisting others to do so, can be difficult. If left uncompleted, however, it can result in unfinished business that may need to be sorted out later on.

As a society of devotees we are blessed with the understanding of the Krishna consciousness philosophy. Daily we strive to increase our devotion to Lord Krishna while simultaneously endeavoring to diminish our attachments to this material world. The process is sublime but requires great determination and effort. Just as we gain strength from the association of other Vaishnavas in our attempt, we also require support from the community of devotees at a time of great loss. Never was this clearer when the following incident occurred.

In the early 1970s, while in the Los Angeles temple, I learned of a godsister who, seemingly without warning, took her own life. Her husband, also an initiated disciple of Srila Prabhupada, was later asked why he moved away from our society of devotees. He replied, "Because my wife committed suicide and no one bothered to ask me how I was feeling."

Obviously, abandonment of a Vaishnava during a time of bereavement can cause devastating hurt and isolation.

Once again we look to Srila Prabhupada for guidance in this matter. After his childhood friend and classmate passed away, Srila Prabhupada wrote in a letter dated September 12, 1976: "Naturally, I am very, very sorry to learn about the death news of your father, my beloved friend. So, offer your mother my condolences for the bereavement, but there is nothing to be very sorry for. According to the *Bhagavad-gita* your father has not died, he has changed his body. *Na hanyate hanyamane sarire* (BG 2.20) Certainly I shall pray to Krishna for his better situation in the next life."

Because losing a friend or family member can be a time of great distress, the bereaved may be eager to hear about the philosophy of Krishna consciousness. Similarly, those who do not practice Krishna consciousness may also become receptive to hearing about the Lord during a time of great sorrow.

In this regard, Srila Prabhupada writes: "When a relative dies one certainly becomes very much interested in philosophy, but when the funeral ceremony is over one again becomes attentive to materialism... The technical term for this attitude of the materialistic person is *smasana-vairagya*, or detachment in a cemetery or place of cremation. As confirmed in *Bhagavad-gita*, four classes of men receive an understanding of spiritual life and God—*arta* (the distressed), *jijnasu* (the inquisitive), *artharthi* (one who desires material gains), and *jnani* (one who is searching for knowledge). Especially when one is very much distressed by material conditions, one becomes interested in God. Therefore, Kuntidevi said in her prayers to Krishna that she preferred distress to a happy mood of life. In the material world, one who is happy forgets Krishna, or God, but sometimes, if one is actually pious but in distress, he remembers Krishna... For a devotee, distress is an opportunity to remember the Supreme Personality of Godhead constantly." (SB 7.2.61)

Naturally, as Vaishnavas, we want to ease the spiritual pain of the bereaved by speaking about the absolute truth, which will ultimately relieve all material distress. But we must be sensitive to their grief and express our compassion for their loss, as exemplified by Srila Prabhupada in the above letter.

Understanding the Grief Reaction

Grief is sometimes described as the emotional reaction to a great loss, while mourning is how one exhibits those feelings of grief. Grieving is a natural process that is necessary in order to heal from the intense feelings of sadness that occur when losing a loved one. Each person will exhibit this sense of loss differently and must evolve in his own way. Therefore, no time restraints or expectations should ever be placed on the bereaved. For some, the amount of grief work to be done after the death of a loved one often depends on how much of the process was worked through prior to the death. Still, a person may experience tremendous emotional struggle when the loss actually occurs.

Other factors affecting the grieving process include the age of the survivor (child, young adult, adult, elderly adult), the cause of the death (longterm painful death, violent accidental death, suicide, peaceful painless death), the nature of the relationship between the bereaved and the deceased, the support system of the bereaved, and the emotional and spiritual health of the person left behind.

Loved ones often express initial feelings of shock and disbelief after months, or even years, of anticipating someone's death. For some, the subsequent grief that is often experienced after losing a dear friend or family member can be one of the most traumatic events in one's life. However, with a significant support system, or even one caring person, the bereaved can emerge from this trauma more emotionally and spiritually healthy. Based on the theories of grief experts such as William Worden, there are three tasks to resolving the loss of someone dear to us. The first task is to understand that the person is actually gone. The second task is to allow one's self to feel the deep emotions that follow such a loss. These feelings may include denial, anger, guilt, fear, and sorrow. The third task of grief is to reinvest in one's life and to connect with others.

There are over seventy signs and symptoms associated with grief that are categorized into feelings, such as fear or guilt or loneliness; thoughts, such as disbelief or confusion; physical sensations, such as tremors or headaches; and behaviors, such as crying or social withdrawal. Again, the grief reaction is individual, but the following time line of critical periods may be helpful when assisting the bereaved to achieve a successful outcome:

- Usually within the first 24-48 hours after a death, the bereaved begin to feel the initial impact of the reality of the death, sometimes simultaneously with a sense of disbelief.

- Mild depression or feelings of sadness, anger, or guilt are often expressed during the first week.

- The most difficult period of adjustment for the bereaved usually occurs within six to eight weeks after a death. Loved ones may begin to feel a sense of loneliness, as the routine of "coming home to an empty house" becomes a reality. Increased depression and anxiety may cause an inability to sleep, weakness and fatigue, mood changes which often include excessive crying, change in eating habits (either lack of interest in food or overeating), confusion, and decreased memory and concentration. A significant event, such as a holiday, may cause the sudden onset of these or other signs and symptoms by one who is grieving a loss.

- A more severe depression may occur approximately six months after the death of a loved one.

- The one-year anniversary of a loved one's death, the birthday of the deceased, a special holiday, or other significant reminder may cause a mild recurrence of depression.

- For some, the bereavement period may continue one to two years or longer after the death of a loved one. Resolution of grief takes place when healthy grief work leads one to fully accept and manage one's loss. Some grief counselors consider the most important grief work to take place up to two years after the death of a loved one.

A Word about Excessive Grief

Excessive grief involves a prolonged, chronic bereavement period in which those experiencing a loss have not successfully progressed through a healthy mourning process. Grief becomes excessive when commonly expressed fears become phobias, when temporary helplessness turns into extended hopelessness, when feelings of guilt become suicidal ideations, and when sadness becomes lingering despair. Early intervention by a professional grief counselor may help to prevent such an extreme situation. If a hospice was involved in caring for the deceased and his family, bereavement support groups and grief counseling is usually offered up to 13 months after a loved one has passed away.

A Word about Insufficient Grief

Many factors may contribute to one's inability to sufficiently grieve, or not grieve at all, after a loss. One's personality, such as intolerance to extreme emotional shifts, or one's unwillingness to admit feelings of vulnerability, even to oneself, may play a significant role. Similarly, a history of multiple losses and the emotional protection that often results can be a contributing factor. Lack of a support system, as well as a social network that diminishes one's loss through awkward silence, may also affect a healthy outcome for the bereaved. With the presence of insufficient grief the bereaved may appear unaffected by his or her loss. Signs and symptoms of grief may appear many years later, however, when triggered by another significant loss. Again, a professional grief counselor can often be of great benefit.

The Tasks of the Bereaved and how We can Help

The bereaved need to accept the reality of their loss. Talking with someone who truly cares about his or her grief can help accomplish this. Denial of one's sorrow does not pave the road to a successful grief outcome; only honest recognition of one's pain can help accomplish this.

How Can We Help? Be patient and listen...and then listen again. Someone who is grieving may repeatedly express the same feelings of disbelief, sadness, frustration, or anger. In such a severe emotional state, verbalization of feelings often requires repetition in order for someone to assimilate his or her sense of loss. As a caregiver, good listening skills can help to unlock a storehouse of grief, which can lead to increased spiritual awareness. If you are accepting of the sense of loss being described, the bereaved will look toward you as a "safe zone," where the most intimate thoughts can be revealed without fear of being judged.

Similarly, you as the caregiver may require expression of your own loss. Seek the shelter of someone who is your "safe zone." You will not be the first caregiver to ever express physical or emotional exhaustion. If you feel guilt or anger, verbalize that as well. *Whatever you are feeling is okay.* As you have just discovered, caring for a terminally ill person is a responsibility that takes its toll on every part of your being. Hopefully, you will have supportive friends and family who can assist you in processing the magnitude of what you have just experienced. Caregivers require nurturing too. Recognize the need to physically, emotionally, and spiritually regenerate. After caring for my mother-in-law for almost a year, I mourned with my relatives for some time after her death and then traveled to Vrindavan with my daughter. After a few weeks in the holy *dhama*, I felt spiritually rejuvenated and was better able to assist my family when we returned home.

The bereaved need to be encouraged to ask for guidance. Often, those who are experiencing a significant loss are not even aware of what they need. Being encouraged to recognize and express what type of help they need from others can assist them in their grieving process as they begin to connect with those who can offer support. In the early stages of grief, practical assistance with everyday tasks may be helpful. Be aware, however, that there can sometimes be a tendency to want to do everything for the one who is in mourning. This is not always the best type of assistance, since learning to live without the deceased is a necessary part of the grief process.

How Can We Help? Never assume what the bereaved need. The only way to know what is needed is to ask. Since those who are grieving can sometimes neglect even their physical needs, encourage proper rest. Offer to bring *prasadam* at various times of the day so those who are mourning do not need to prepare their own meals. This simple act of kindness will convey a strong message of caring. In addition, numerous details at this time can seem overwhelming. Offer to help with funeral arrangements, make phone calls, send emails, or assist with sorting through legal and financial paperwork. Provide transportation if needed. Even the simplest of chores may feel like an effort for those who are grieving. If young children are involved, offer to assist with their care, especially within the first week or so after the death. Remember that children need to grieve as well. They need answers to their questions and reinforcement that remaining loved ones will not leave them at this crucial time. When a family member dies, it will naturally affect the way the family functions as a whole. Relationships within the family may shift, adjusting to change in the family structure. Young children and adolescents may mourn for the family that no longer exists.

Being an empathetic listener is often the best way to assist the bereaved. (There is no need to offer advice unless you are asked.) Unless it is a necessity, it is recommended that change of residence be avoided for at least six months to a year after the death of a loved one. The stress that accompanies grief often causes difficulty with sound, objective decision-making. If reasonable, encourage those who are grieving to postpone making major decisions at this time. Independent decision-making, beginning with smaller issues, should be encouraged as one progresses in his or her healing.

The bereaved need to share their memories. To reminisce is to honor the departed Vaishnava. Sharing memories may give a new perspective to one's loss as well as help the bereaved to adjust to a life in which a loved one is no longer present.

How Can We Help? Ask to see photographs or videos. Ask questions about the deceased to encourage a discussion. Recall your own memories, and express the difference it made in your life to have known the departed Vaishnava. Take their lead, however. When they are ready, the bereaved will share their memories, if that is what is needed for recovery. Discussions such as this should never be forced. They will naturally develop in time.

The bereaved need our honesty. It is never easy to console those who are grieving. It is not uncommon to be at a loss for words. Sometimes if we admit our discomfort and feelings of helplessness to the bereaved, we will feel at ease with the silence that often accompanies their sorrow.

How Can We Help? It is appropriate to say something like, "I wish I knew what to say or do to take your pain away. Please know that I am here for you, though." Avoid cliches such as, "I know how you feel." Even if we have experienced a similar loss, it is difficult to know exactly how someone else feels. Saying "Try to be strong" is of little comfort at this time. Sometimes your quiet presence may be more helpful than anything you can say. Nonverbal messages, such as holding a hand or a gentle touch on the shoulder, can often communicate a greater sense of caring than any words we can express.

The bereaved need continued support. Often within a week or two of the funeral service, friends and family return to their usual routines, leaving the bereaved to cope with their pain alone. We can never measure the depth of someone else's emotional wound. A kind gesture at this time can give great comfort and ease loneliness.

How Can We Help? Provide a "lifeline" by letting the bereaved know they can call you at any time. Call them as well. Send a note just to let them know you are thinking about them. Offer to visit. The association of devotees can provide great spiritual strength. Offer to accompany them to a temple for *darshan* of the Deities. Suggest taking quiet walks together. Chant the Hare Krishna *mantra* together. Offer to read aloud Srila Prabhupada's books. Continue to listen and to reaffirm your support. Provide a nurturing environment to help promote a healthy resolution to the loss. Listen for statements that may indicate the need for "permission" to stop grieving and to move on with their lives.

Rejoicing for the Departed Vaishnava

He reasons ill who tells that Vaishnavas die
When thou art living still in sound.
The Vaishnavas die to live, and living try
To spread the holy name around
　　　　　　　　　　　　　　　　—Srila Bhaktivinode Thakur

Although it is natural to feel continued separation from a loved one, those who are working through their grief are free to simultaneously search for spiritual meaning to their loss. The transcendental knowledge contained in Srila Prabhupada's books can provide us with the spiritual answers we need to eventually feel at peace with the auspicious departure of the Lord's devotee. Ultimately, engaging in the nine processes of devotional service—hearing about the Lord, chanting His holy names, remembering the Lord, worshiping the Lord, serving the lotus feet of the Lord, offering prayers, carrying out the orders of the Lord, making friends with Him, and surrendering everything to the Lord, as prescribed in Srila Prabhupada's *Bhagavad-gita As It Is*—can relieve one from the most severe type of material distress. The following instruction from Srila Prabhupada's *Nectar of Devotion*, for example, has comforted me during times of great loss within my own life. Srila Prabhupada writes:

> In the Tenth Canto, Fourteenth Chapter, Verse 8, it is said, 'My dear Lord, any person who is constantly awaiting Your causeless mercy to be bestowed upon him, and who goes on suffering the resultant actions of his past misdeeds, offering You respectful obeisances from the core of his heart, is surely eligible to become liberated, for it has become his rightful claim.' This statement of *Srimad-Bhagavatam* should be the guide of all devotees. A devotee should not expect immediate relief from the reactions of his past misdeeds... A devotee who is not perfectly freed from the resultant actions should therefore continue to act in Krishna consciousness seriously, even though there may be so many impediments. When such impediments arise, he should simply think of Krishna and expect His mercy. That is the only solace. If the devotee passes his days in this spirit, it is certain that he is going to be promoted to the abode of the Lord. By such activities, he earns his claim to enter into the kingdom of God.

Indeed, the healing words of a pure devotee of the Lord can soothe one's turbulent mind and steady one's wavering faith.

Additional Quotations from Srila Prabhupada

When the bereaved are receptive to hearing them, the following are some quotations from Srila Prabhupada's books that can uplift one from a distraught position to one of spiritual understanding. Srila Prabhupada's writings can console one who is grieving any type of loss within this material world, what to speak of easing one's separation from a beloved Vaishnava who has departed from this world.

> And in due course of time, when a pure devotee is completely prepared, all of a sudden the change of body occurs which is commonly

called death. And for the pure devotee such a change takes place exactly like lightning, and illumination follows simultaneously. That is to say a devotee simultaneously changes his material body and develops a spiritual body by the will of the Supreme. (SB 1.6.27)

The preliminary instruction in the *Bhagavad-gita* is that one should know that the identity of the individual living entity is not lost even after the end of this present body, which is nothing but an outward dress only. As one changes an old garment, so the individual living being also changes his body, and this change of body is called death. Death is therefore a process of changing the body at the end of the duration of the present life. An intelligent person must be prepared for this and must try to have the best type of body in the next life. The best type of body is a spiritual body, which is obtained by those who go back to the kingdom of God or enter the realm of *Brahman*. (SB 2.1.15)

If one can remember Krishna at death, he is immediately transferred to Goloka Vrindavan, or Krsnaloka, and thus his life becomes successful. (SB 4.23.13)

The Lord says in *Bhagavad-gita* (8.5):

anta-kale ca mam eva
smaran muktva kalevaram
yah prayati sa mad-bhavam
yati nasty atra samsayah

Whoever, at the time of death, quits his body remembering Me alone at once attains My nature. Of this there is no doubt.

Of course, one must practice before one is overcome by death, but the perfect *yogi*, namely the devotee, dies in trance, thinking of Krishna. He does not feel his material body being separated from his soul; the soul is immediately transferred to the spiritual world. *Tyaktva deham punar janma naiti mam eti*: the soul does not enter the womb of a material mother again, but is transferred back home, back to Godhead... The *bhakti-yogi* always thinks of Krishna, and therefore at the time of death he can very easily transfer himself to Krsnaloka, without even perceiving the pains of death. (SB 6.10.12)

The *Padma Purana* also mentions, 'A person whose body is decorated with the pulp of sandalwood, with paintings of the holy name of the Lord, is delivered from all sinful reactions, and after his death he goes directly to Krsnaloka to live in association with the Supreme Personality of Godhead.' (*Nectar of Devotion*)

Even if devotees are illusioned by some ghastly scene or by any accidental occurrence, they never forget Krishna. Even in the greatest danger they can remember Krishna. This is the benefit of Krishna consciousness: even at the time of death, when all the functions of the body become dislocated, the devotee can remember Krishna in his innermost consciousness, and this saves him from falling down into material existence. In this way Krishna consciousness immediately takes one from the material platform to the spiritual world. (*Nectar of Devotion*)

Some way or other, if someone establishes in his mind his continuous relationship with Krishna, this relationship is called remembrance. About this remembrance there is a nice statement in the *Visnu Purana*, where it is said, 'Simply by remembering the Supreme Personality of Godhead all living entities become eligible for all kinds of auspiciousness. Therefore let me always remember the Lord, who is unborn and eternal.' In the *Padma Purana* the same remembrance is explained as follows: 'Let me offer my respectful obeisances unto the Supreme Lord Krishna, because if someone remembers Him, either at the time of death or during his span of life, he becomes freed from all sinful reactions.' (*Nectar of Devotion*)

Anyone who quits his body in Krishna consciousness is at once transferred to the transcendental abode of the Supreme Lord... To remember Krishna one should chant the *maha-mantra*, Hare Krishna, Hare Krishna, Krishna Krishna, Hare Hare, Hare Rama, Hare Rama, Rama Rama, Hare Hare, incessantly, following in the footsteps of Lord Chaitanya, being more tolerant than the tree, humbler than the grass and offering all respect to others without requiring respect in return. In such a way one will be able to depart from the body successfully remembering Krishna and so attain the supreme goal. (BG 8.5)

By chanting Krishna's names, one will be transferred to the supreme planet, Krsnaloka, without a doubt. (BG 8.7)

To a devotee who is thus engaged in Krishna consciousness the Lord is very, very kind. In spite of all difficulties, he is eventually placed in the transcendental abode, or Krsnaloka. He is guaranteed entrance there; there is no doubt about it. In that supreme abode, there is no change; everything is eternal, imperishable, and full of knowledge. (BG 18.56)

After the death of his dear disciple, Jayananda Das, Srila Prabhupada wrote the following letter on May 5, 1977:

My dear Jayananda,

Please accept my blessings. I am feeling very intensely your separation. In 1967 you joined me in San Francisco. You were driving my car and chanting Hare Krishna. You were the first man to give me some contribution ($5,000) for printing my *Bhagavad-gita*. After that, you have rendered very favorable service to Krishna in different ways. I so hope at the time of your death you were remembering Krishna and as such, you have been promoted to the eternal association of Krishna. If not, if you had any tinge of material desire, you have gone to the celestial kingdom to live with the demigods for many thousands of years and enjoy the most opulent life of material existence. From there you can promote yourself to the spiritual world. But even if one fails to promote oneself to the spiritual world, at that time he comes down again on the surface of this globe and takes birth in a big family like *yogis* or *brahmanas* or an aristocratic family, where there is again a chance of reviving Krishna consciousness. But, as you were hearing Krishna-kirtana, I am sure that you were directly promoted to Krishnaloka.

> *janma karma ca me divyam*
> *evam yo vetti tattvatah*
> *tyaktva deham punar janma*
> *naiti mam eti so'rjuna*
>
> (BG 4.9)

Krishna has done a great favor to you, not to continue your diseased body, and has given you a suitable place for your service. Thank you very much.

Your ever well-wisher, A.C. Bhaktivedanta Swami

Concluding Words

> *After many births and deaths, he who is actually in knowledge surrenders unto Me, knowing Me to be the cause of all causes and all that is. Such a great soul is very rare.*
>
> (BG 7.19)

One who lives in the association of the Lord's devotees is most fortunate, but one who truly appreciates that association has a blessed life. Out of billions of people on this earth, only a tiny percentage know Krishna to be God, and out of those, only a handful recognize Srila Prabhupada's contribution to the world by bringing Krishna consciousness to the West.

Every soul who comes to our Krishna consciousness movement is precious. As a society of devotees engaged in the service of His Divine Grace, we need to care for one another in every stage of life. Since there is no time more important to a Vaishnava than the moment of death, a devotee should not have to spend his or her final days alone in a hospital or nursing home without the association of other Vaishnavas. Certainly, a special soul who has given so much of his or her life to the Lord deserves to be given the holy names when dying. My hope is that I have conveyed this message within the pages of this book and in some small way inspired its readers to assist others with the final journey back home, back to Godhead.

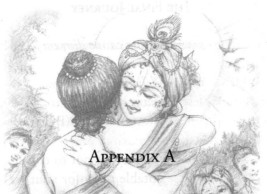

Appendix A

Procedure for Placing Ashes in the Yamuna River

by Deena Bandhu Das

Requirements:

1. A picture of the departed person
2. Pictures of Radha-Krishna, Gaura-Nitai, and Srila Prabhupada
3. Arati tray with the following items:
   a Ghee lamp and wick (wicks can be purchased at the *ghat*)
   b Bell
   c *Achman* cup and spoon
   d A small pack of incense
   e Matches/lighter (Here in Vrindavan it is recommended to have lots of matches since we are on the river. Sometimes in the rainy season they don't light very well and there is sometimes a breeze to make things difficult!)
4. A couple of *bhoga* garlands and flowers (not offered yet to the deities)
5. Option of *prasad* garlands to offer to the departed (already offered to the Deities)
6. *Bhoga* sweets (not offered yet to the Lord). I usually recommend a good variety just to make it nice, two pieces each of several different kinds. A kilo is sufficient, depending on how many people are participating.
7. *Tulasi* leaves (Many times the ladies who sell the wicks at the *ghat* also have these.)

8. A few leaf cups or something similar for making the offering
9. Cloth for bathing
10. A nice cloth for setting up the altar
11. Some of the black plastic boxes the ashes come in are sealed and you may need a knife to open it. (I always carry a Swiss army knife with me!)
12. Some copies of the *Yamunastakam* prayers so that everyone can participate.

Procedure:

Ordinarily we do this ceremony in the morning after breakfast so that more devotees can attend. It should take a couple of hours so that the ceremony is completed around noon, at which time everyone bathes in the Yamuna river.

We pick a nicely decorated boat, with a covering for shade if the weather is hot. We will end up paying around Rs500 as theoretically they have to wash their whole boat down afterwards, and also because at such a time we don't want to get into a nasty argument over price! On the back of the boat there is a platform for making a nice altar. With my fold-up altar we wedge it between the platform and the back of the boat when it is windy. If there is no frame for the picture of the departed, the same applies. The departed's picture is put on the left side of the altar.

Then we leisurely float down the Yamuna with the devotees having *kirtan*. We light several sticks of incense and place them around the boat, being careful to place them where no one can accidentally burn their cloth. First we offer the *bhoga* garlands to the Deity pictures. Some of each of the sweets are put into leaf cups and an offering is made. After offering the sweets, we move the *mahaprasad* in front of the departed's picture, as well as one of the garlands that was offered to the Deity pictures, and then the *mahaprasad* is offered to the deceased person. After offering the *mahaprasad*, we then beg permission from Sri Yamunaji for putting the ashes in her waters by carefully floating a couple of leaf cups with a little *mahaprasad*. A ghee wick can optionally be offered on top. Then, again to pacify Sri Yamunaji, we chant the *Yamunasthakam* of Srila Rupa Goswami.

We continue the *kirtan* by chanting the Hare Krishna *maha mantra*. We usually go to the other shore and those who are placing the ashes in the Yamuna change into their bathing cloth. Most of the time, there is an urn or a black plastic box with the ashes. We wade into the water up to our thighs. None of the ashes should go into the air, so the container has to be immersed into the water completely and water allowed to enter to mix with the ashes. In the case of an urn or pot with no plastic bag, the mouth has to be covered and immersed in the water and water slowly allowed to enter. Then the ashes are released in the waters of the Yamuna river while the others throw flowers and the flower garlands over the water. Then everyone takes a bath and with *kirtan*, we return to the opposite shore.

Depending on the means it is nice to offer a feast for the Vaishnavas after the ceremony. This can be held at the temple or wherever is practical. In addition, many devotees choose to sponsor a feast for elderly widows who reside in the *dham*. In lieu of a feast, you can offer some sweets to the devotees. It is also recommended to make a donation to the cows in the *dham*, so after the ceremony you can make an affordable donation to the Krishna-Balaram Goshalla (ISKCON's cow protection project).

Sri Yamunastakam

by Srila Rupa Goswami

1   *bhratur antakasya pattane 'bhipatti-harini*
    preksayati-papino 'pi papa-sindhu-tarini
    nira-madhuribhir apy asesa-citta-bandhini
    mam punatu sarvadaravinda-bandhu-nandini

"May Yamunadevi, the daughter of Suryadeva, always purify me. She saves all who touch her from going to the realm of her brother Yamaraja, and enables even greatly wicked persons, who see her, to cross the ocean of their sinful deeds. Her attractive water charms the hearts of everyone."

2   *hari-vari-dharayabhimanditoru-khandava*
    pundarika-mandalodyad-andajali-tandava

snana-kama-pamarogra-papa-sampad-andhini
mam punatu sarvadaravinda-bandhu-nandini

"Yamunadevi adorns Indra's great Khandava forest with her enchanting current, and upon her blooming lotus flowers various birds are always dancing. Simply desiring to bathe in her pleasant, crystalline waters frees one from even the greatest of sins. May Yamunadevi, the daughter of Suryadeva, always purify me."

3   *sikarabhimrista-jantu-durvipaka-mardini*
       nanda-nandanantaranga-bhakti-pura-vardhini
       tira-sangamabhilasi-mangalanubandhini
       mam punatu sarvadaravinda-bandhu-nandini

"Sprinkling a single drop of her water upon oneself destroys the reaction of the most heinous crimes. She increases the flow of confidential devotional service (*raganuga-bhakti*) for Nandanandana within one's heart and blesses everyone who simply desires to reside on her banks. May Yamunadevi, the daughter of Suryadeva, always purify me."

4   *dvipa-cakravala-justa-sapta-sindhu-bhedini*
       sri-mukunda-nirmitoru-divya-keli-vedini
       kanti-kandalibhir indranila-vrinda-nindini
       mam punatu sarvadaravinda-bandhu-nandini

"Yamunadevi is so powerful, that although she flows through the seven oceans which surround the earth's seven islands, she never merges with them. Being witness to many of Sri Mukunda's wonderful pastimes, she manifests these pastimes in the hearts of those who take shelter of her. Her dark, shimmering beauty defeats the splendor of precious blue sapphires. May Yamunadevi, the daughter of Suryadeva, always purify me."

5   *mathurena mandalena carunabhimandita*
       prema-naddha-vaisnavadhva-vardhanaya pandita
       urmi-dor-vilasa-padmanabha-pada-vandini
       mam punatu sarvadaravinda-bandhu-nandini

"Ornamented with the supremely enchanting land of Mathura-mandala, Yamunadevi skillfully inspires love of Godhead (*prema*) in the hearts of the Vaishnavas who bathe in her. With playful waves, which are like her moving arms, she worships Padmanabha Sri Krishna's lotus feet. May Yamunadevi, the daughter of Suryadeva, always purify me."

6   *ramya-tira-rambhamana-go-kadamba-bhusita*
divya-gandha-bhak-kadamba-puspa-raji-rusita
nanda-sunu-bhakta-sangha-sangamabhinandini
mam punatu sarvadaravinda-bandhu-nandini

"Yamunadevi's charming banks are further beautified by the fragrance from the flowers of *kadamba* trees and by loving cows. She is especially delighted when Nandalala's devotees assemble on her banks. May Yamunadevi, the daughter of Suryadeva, always purify me."

7   *phulla-paksa-mallikaksa-hamsa-laksa-kujita*
bhakti-viddha-deva-siddha-kinnarali-pujita
tira-gandhavaha-gandha-janma-bandha-randhini
mam punatu sarvadaravinda-bandhu-nandini

"Filled with the warbling of thousands of joyful swans, Yamunadevi is worshipable to demigods, Siddhas, Kinnaras and humans whose hearts are dedicated to the service of Sri Hari. Anyone who is touched by her gentle breezes is freed from the cycle of birth and death. May Yamunadevi, the daughter of Suryadeva, always purify me."

8   *cid-vilasa-vari-pura-bhur-bhuvah-svar-apini*
kirtitapi durmadoru-papa-marma-tapini
ballavendra-nandanangaraga-bhanga-gandhini
mam punatu sarvadaravinda-bandhu-nandini

"Yamunadevi flows through the three worlds known as Bhuh, Bhuvah and Svah and distributes her loving emotions. Singing her glories burns even the greatest sins to ashes. She has become fragrant by the scented ointments from the body of King Nanda's son Sri Krishna, who enjoys to play in her waters. May Yamunadevi, the daughter of Suryadeva, always purify me."

9   *tusta-buddhir astakena nirmalormi-cestitam*
tvam anena bhanu-putri sarva-deva-vestitam
yah staviti vardhayasva sarva-papa-mocane
bhakti-puram asya devi pundarika-locane

"O Suryaputri! Devi! O Yamuna, whose waves are very purifying and who is surrounded by all the demigods! For those who recite with cheerful heart these prayers, please increase their bhakti for lotus-eyed Sri Krishna, who liberates all persons from their sins."

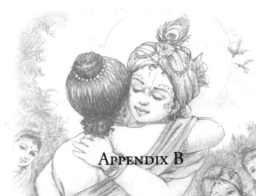

Appendix B

Procedure for Placing Ashes in the Ganges River

by Jananivas Das

Articles required:
1. Cow dung
2. Cow Urine
3. Ghee
4. Milk
5. Yogurt
6. Barley seeds
7. Chandan paste
8. Flowers
9. Banana
10. Sesame seeds (white til)
11. Kusa grass (3 pieces with roots and tips intact)
12. Bamboo plate or clay pot
13. Copper vessel
14. Honey
15. Kusa grass tips

Make Pancha Gavya
Mix the following ingredients in equal proportions in the following order:
1. Kusa grass tips
2. Cow dung (diluted in water)
3. Cow urine

4. Ghee (melt ghee if solid)
5. Yogurt
6. Milk

Smear the bamboo plate with clay. (If the ashes are less in quantity then the following procedure can be done in a clay cup made from the available clay there on the banks.)

Put the following ingredients in this order in the bamboo plate:
1. Ashes
2. Pancha gavya
3. Barley seeds
4. White til
5. Honey

Then cover it completely with clay from the Ganges.

Take bath in the Ganges.

Loosen the knot of shikha and shift the Brahmin thread to the right shoulder while taking bath. After taking bath shift the Brahmin thread back to the left shoulder and tie the shikha and perform arcaman.

Fill the copper vessel with Ganges water then put the following ingredients in it:
1. Sesame seeds
2. Flowers
3. Peeled banana
4. 3 pc kusa grass with root and tip intact

Chant brahma gayatri mantra 10 times over the water then perform Matsya Mudra.

Offer flower puspanjali to Gangadevi.
Esa puspanjali om gangaya namah

Sankalpa
Face north and chant the following mantras:
1. Chant one's Guru Maharaja's pranam mantra
2. Srila Prabhupada's pranam mantra

Procedure for Placing Ashes in the Ganges River

3. Namo Mahavadanyaya………..
4. Namo Brahmanya………………..
5. Jai Sri Krishna Chaitanya…………
6. Hare Krishna Hare Krishna………..
7. Vishnu om tat sat
8. Govinda Govinda Govinda

Specify the day of the year on which the ceremony is being performed. This can be obtained from the local Panjika or Pandit or ISKCON's calendar available from the internet.

Asya:

_____Gaurabdha (year, ie number of years after 1486)
_____Masa (lunar month)
_____Paksha
(Light or dark fortnight. Gaura Paksha or Krishna Paksha)
_____Yoga (time)
_____Nakshatra (star)
_____Tithi (lunar day)
_____Gotra (Acyuta gotra for all Vaishnavas)
_____Name of the deceased

Sri Krishna prityartha etany asthini gangayam viniksipami karmaham karisye
Hare Krishna Hare Krishna………..

Place right hand over the left and receive water from the copper pot in the hand and release the water in North East direction (do this 3 times).

Turn the copper pot upside down and put flowers and chandan on the top.

Then recite the sankalpa sukta (Yajur Veda):
Om yaj jagrato duram udaiti daivam tad u suptasya tathaivaiti Durangamam jyotisam jyotirekam tan me manah siva sankalpam astu Hare Krishna Hare Krishna …………..

Take the ashes and enter into the waters of Mother Ganga.
Chant the following mantra:
Om namastu dharmaya
Go as far as possible and then consign the ashes to Gangadevi.
Chant:
Om saha me prito bhavatu—If the deceased was male
Om sa me prito bhavatu—If the deceased was female

Take a dip in the Ganges and perform tarpan for the eternal family.

Mantras for doing tarpan:
While standing in the Ganga, face east, take water from the Ganga in cupped hands and pour into the Ganga over the fingertips for each of the following mantras:

om guruve tarpayami
om para guruve tarpayami
om para para guruve tarpayami
om maha guruve tarpayami
om paramesthi guruve tarpayami
om sarva vaishnavabhyo tarpayami
om sarva vaishnavibhyo tarpayami
om sri pancatattva tarpayami
om sri sri radha krishna tarpayami

For the deceased:
Facing southwards, take Ganga water in both hands and with sesame seeds added, chant:

Om Visnu
Om tat sat
Gotra
Pitra/matra (if father or mother)
Name of deceased
Etat satila gango dakam tubham swadha

After chanting the mantras, open the right thumb, pour the water

Procedure for Placing Ashes in the Ganges River

from the right side of the hand between the thumb and forefinger. Repeat three times.

Then chant Hare Krishna Hare Krishna................

Take dip in Mother Ganges and give remuneration to the priest and offer prasadam to at least one brahmana.

Please note that there may be minor changes in the details according to different customs in different locations.

<u>**Chanting Hare Krishna Mahamantra and distribution of prasadam are the two most important items.**</u>

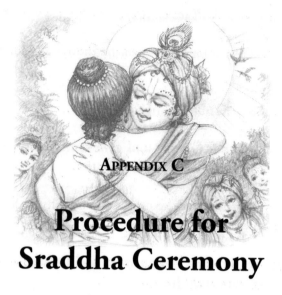

Appendix C

Procedure for Sraddha Ceremony

by Jananivas Das

Articles required:
1. Chandan paste
2. Flowers
3. 1 Banana
4. Sesame seeds (white til)
5. Kusa grass (3 pieces with roots and tips intact)
6. Copper vessel
7. 2 plates of Mahaprasad

1. Take bath in the Ganges.

Loosen the knot of the shikha and shift the Brahmin thread to the right shoulder while taking bath. After taking bath shift the Brahmin thread back to the left shoulder, tie the shikha and perform arcaman.

2. From the river bank, fill the copper vessel with Ganges water and then put the following ingredients in it:
   a. Sesame seeds
   b. Flowers
   c. Peeled banana
   d. 3 pc kusa grass with root and tip intact

Procedure for Sraddha Ceremony

Chant gayatri mantra over the water while performing Matsya Mudra.

3. Offer one plate of Mahaprasad and flower puspanjali to Gangadevi.
Idam mahaprasadam om gangaya namah
Esa puspanjali om gangaya namah

4. Sankalpa
Face north and chant the following mantras:
a. Chant one's Guru Maharaja's Pranam mantra.
b. Srila Prabhupada's pranam mantra
c. *Namo Mahavadanyaya...........*
d. *Namo Brahmanya....................*
e. *Jai Sri Krishna Chaitanya............*
f. *Hare Krishna Hare Krishna...........*
g. *Vishnu om tat sat*
h. *Govinda Govinda Govinda*

Specify the day of the year on which the ceremony is being performed. This can be obtained from the local Panjika or Pandit or ISKCON's calendar available from the internet.

Asya:

_____Gaurabdha (year, ie number of years after 1486)
_____Masa (lunar month)
_____Paksha
(Light or dark fortnight. Gaura Paksha or Krishna Paksha)
_____Yoga (time)
_____Nakshatra (star)
_____Tithi (lunar day)
_____Gotra (Acyuta gotra for all Vaishnavas)
_____Name of the deceased

Sri Krishna prityartha etany asthini gangayam viniksipami karmaham karisye
Hare Krishna Hare Krishna...........

Place right hand over the left and receive water from the copper pot in the hand and release the water in North East direction (do this 3 times).

Turn the copper pot upside down and put flowers and chandan on the top.

Then recite the sankalpa sukta (Yajur Veda):
Om yaj jagrato duram udaiti daivam tad u suptasya tathaivaiti
Durangamam jyotisam jyotirekam tan me manah siva sankalpam astu
Hare Krishna Hare Krishna ....

5. Take a dip in the Ganges and perform tarpan for the eternal family.

Mantras for doing tarpan
While standing in the Ganga, face east, take water from the Ganga in cupped hands and pour into the Ganga over the finger tips, for each of the following mantras:

om guruve tarpayami
om para guruve tarpayami
om para para guruve tarpayami
om maha guruve tarpayami
om paramesthi guruve tarpayami
om sarva vaishnavabhyo tarpayami
om sarva vaishnavibhyo tarpayami
om sri pancatattva tarpayami
om sri sri radha krishna tarpayami

For the deceased:
Facing southwards, take Ganga water in both hands and with sesame seeds added, chant:

Om Visnu
Om tat sat
Gotra
Pitra/matra (if father or mother)

Name of deceased
Etat satila gango dakam tubham swadha
After chanting the mantras, open the right thumb; pour the water from the right side of the hand between the thumb and forefinger.

Repeat three times.

Then chant Hare Krishna Hare Krishna................

6. Take dip in Mother Ganges and give remuneration to the priest and offer prasadam to at least one brahmana.

Please note that there may be minor changes in the details according to different customs in different locations.

<u>Chanting Hare Krishna Mahamantra and distribution of prasadam are the two most important items.</u>

Glossary

A

Acharya—A spiritual instructor who teaches by example and who is in an authorized line of disciplic succession.

Adjuvant—A drug that is added to a prescription to increase the action of the principal ingredient, or to speed its onset of action.

Amyotrophic Lateral Sclerosis—ALS. A syndrome caused by degeneration of nerve cells in the spinal cord. Symptoms are muscular weakness and atrophy (wasting away of the muscles), contractions of the muscles causing awkward movements, and increased actions of reflexes.

Analgesic—a drug that is given to relieve pain.

Anemia—Low number of circulating red blood cells. Hemoglobin, the iron-containing component of the red blood cell, is less than that needed to supply the body's oxygen demand. This may be caused by excessive blood loss, excessive blood cell destruction, or a decrease in blood cell formation.

Angiogram—Serial X-rays taken in rapid sequence following the injection of a substance that is impenetrable to X-rays or other forms of radiation. In this way, the size and shape of various veins and arteries of organs and tissues can be defined.

Anorexia—Loss of appetite; may be caused by a variety of problems such as disorders of the stomach, depression, malaise, fever, illnesses, or medications.

Antagonist—That which counteracts the action of something else. A narcotic antagonist is a drug that prevents or reverses the action of a narcotic.

Antibodies—Protein substances that develop in the body in response to an antigen (a substance that may be introduced into, or may form within, the body). Antibodies may be present due to previous infection, vaccination, transfer from mother to fetus in utero, or an unknown antigen stimulus.

Anticonvulsant—An agent that prevents or relieves convulsion (involuntary contraction and relaxation of muscles).

Antiemetic—An agent that prevents or relieves nausea and vomiting.
Anti-inflammatory—An agent that counteracts inflammation.
Antipyretic—An agent that reduces fever.
Antiseptic—A substance that stops or slows the growth or action of microorganisms.
Apnea—The periodic, transient stopping of respirations.
Arjuna—Lord Krishna's dear friend and devotee to whom He spoke the *Bhagavad-gita* on the battlefield of Kurukshetra.
Arati—A worship ceremony in which the Lord in His Deity form is offered lamps and other items of devotion.
Arrhythmia—Irregular heart beat.
Ashram—1) A basic living quarter in a temple or holy place conducive to spiritual life. 2) Vedic social system with four spiritual orders of life: *brahmacarya* (student life), *grihastha* (married life), *vanaprastha* (retired life), and *sannyasa* (renounced order of life).
Aspiration—Drawing in or out as by suction. Foreign bodies may be aspirated into the nose, throat, or lungs upon inhalation.
Autoimmune response—Production of antibodies, or T cells (white blood cells that help with immunity) that attack a person's own tissues.

B

Bhagavad-gita—Literally means "song of God." The Supreme Personality of Godhead, Lord Sri Krishna, instructs his disciple Arjuna about devotional service and spiritual life in this sacred scripture.
Bhajan—Worshiping God, or His pure devotee, through music and song.
Bhakti-yoga—A process of linking with the Supreme Lord by devotional service to Him.
Brahmacari—A celibate student; the first of the four Vedic *ashrams*.
Bhoga—Food not yet offered to the Lord.
Brijbasi—A resident of the holy land of Vrindavan, India.
Bronchitis—Inflammation of the bronchi, which are the two main branches leading from the trachea to the lungs. These provide a passageway for air movement.
Bronchodilator—A medication that causes dilation of the bronchus (windpipe).

C

CHF—See "congestive heart failure."

CNS—See "central nervous system."

CT—See "computerized or computed tomography."

Cardiac catheterization—A diagnostic procedure used to determine heart disorders and anomalies. A tiny plastic tube is passed into the heart through a blood vessel. Samples of blood are withdrawn for examination; blood pressure and the amount of blood the heart pumps per minute are measured.

Caranamrita—The water that remains after bathing the feet of the Deity of the Lord.

Cellulitis—Inflammation of cellular or connective tissue, causing redness, swelling, and if severe, weeping of fluid through the skin.

Central nervous system—CNS. Includes the brain and spinal cord along with their nerves and end organs that control voluntary actions.

Cerebral cortex—The outer gray area of the cerebrum (the largest part of the brain).

Cerebrospinal fluid—Watery, clear, colorless fluid that acts as a cushion protecting the brain and spinal cord from physical impact. A small amount of this fluid can be extracted and examined for diagnostic purposes.

Chaitanya Mahaprabhu—Lord Krishna Himself who came to this earth in the form of a devotee. He appeared in West Bengal in the late 15th century and inaugurated the congregational chanting of the holy names of the Lord as the means for self-realization in this present age.

Chemoreceptor trigger zone—A sensory nerve ending, or nerve organ, that reacts to particular chemical stimuli, and is located outside of the central nervous system.

Chemotherapy—The treatment of disease, especially cancer, by the use of various drugs designed to destroy abnormal cells.

Cheyne-Stokes respirations—Apnea (transient cessation of breathing), followed by increasing depth and frequency of respirations.

Cirrhosis—A chronic disease of the liver characterized by an overgrowth of tissue or fibroses (overgrowth of fibrous connective tissue called scar tissue).

Computerized or computed tomography—CT. A refined version of X-ray equipment. As the patient's body is slowly moved through the doughnut-shaped CT machine, the X-ray tube around the body sends beams to a specific level of the patient's body. In this way, thin slices of the body can be viewed, eliminating the confusion resulting from overlapping structures seen in conventional X-rays.

Compression stockings—Stockings made of stretch material that maintains pressure against the legs and reduces swelling.

Congestive heart failure—CHF. A condition characterized by breathlessness, weakness, swelling in the lower portions of the body and abdominal discomfort. This results from the inability of the heart to pump effectively, causing blood circulation to be inadequate to meet the body's needs.

Continuous oxygen therapy—The continuous administration of oxygen for the treatment of conditions resulting from a deficiency of oxygen. Continuous oxygen is usually administered at home by nasal cannula (plastic tubing leading from the oxygen tank to the patient with two small outlet prongs that are inserted into the nostrils).

Continuous subcutaneous infusion—A continuous infusion, by use of a pump, of a substance into the tissue just beneath the skin.

Corticosteroid—A hormonal steroid medication.

Cystic fibrosis—CF. A disease that is inherited and affects the pancreas, respiratory system, and sweat glands. It is characterized by chronic respiratory infections, heat intolerance, and insufficient pancreas function. The prognosis is poor and there is presently no cure.

CPR—Cardiopulmonary resuscitation. The process used to attempt to restore normal breathing and heartbeat when these have stopped. This procedure includes clearing air passages, "breathing" air into the lungs, heart massage, and sometimes drugs.

D

DKA—See "diabetic ketoacidosis."
DNA—See "deoxyribonucleic acid."
Darshan—Viewing of the Deity of the Lord.
Decoction—The result of the process of extracting the flavor or essence of a substance by boiling.

Decubitus ulcer—An ulcer commonly caused by pressure to an area of the body from a bed or chair. Measured according to severity as Stage I-IV.

Deity—A statue worshiped in a temple or home as a representation of the personal form of God.

Deoxyribonucleic acid—DNA. Found in all living cells and carries the organism's hereditary information.

Dharma—Religious principles.

Diabetes mellitus—A disorder of carbohydrate metabolism, characterized by abnormally high amounts of glucose (sugar) in the blood and urine, and resulting from improper utilization or inadequate production of insulin.

Diabetic ketoacidosis—A serious disorder that can be life-threatening. When sugars cannot be used by the body's cells as fuel, more fats are mobilized resulting in high fatty acid levels in the blood. Ketones are formed from these fatty acids, which are strong organic acids. When they accumulate faster than they are used or excreted, the blood pH drops resulting in ketoacidosis.

Diabetic neuropathy—A common complication of diabetes, in which nerves are damaged as a result of high blood sugar levels.

Diuretic—A medication that increases the amount of urine secreted.

Dopamine—A substance synthesized by the adrenal glands (located on each kidney) that acts to increase blood pressure and urine output.

Dysphagia—Difficulty or inability to swallow.

E

EEG—See "electroencephalogram."

EKG—See "electrocardiogram."

Echocardiogram—A diagnostic process that uses ultrasound in order to visualize the internal structures of the heart.

Edema—Generalized or localized swelling; a condition in which the body tissues contain an abnormally large amount of fluid. Often edema is seen in dependent areas (parts of the body lower than the heart), but may present anywhere in the body.

Electrocardiogram—ECG, EKG. A record of wave patterns showing the electrical activity of the heart. Evaluation of these wave patterns is instrumental in diagnosing cardiac abnormalities.

Electroencephalogram—EEG. A tracing of brain waves made by an electroencephalograph that records the electrical activity of the brain. Evaluation of these tracings is instrumental in diagnosing various diseases and localizing brain tumors.

Electrolyte—A substance that, in solution, conducts an electric current. There are several electrolytes in the blood, interstitial fluid, and intercellular fluid of the body. It is important for these electrolytes to stay in a constant balance for proper body function.

Electromyogram—A graphic recording of muscle contractions used for diagnostic purposes.

Electromyography—The study of electromyograms.

Embolism—A foreign substance, generally a blood clot, causing an obstruction in a blood vessel.

Emphysema—A chronic lung disease, of which the most characteristic sign is breathlessness upon exertion.

Endocarditis—Inflammation of the lining of the heart that could be caused by bacteria or an abnormal immune response.

Endorphins—A group of proteins that occur naturally in the brain and have potent analgesic properties.

Enteric-coated—A tablet or capsule coated with a special compound that will not dissolve until it is in contact with the fluids in the small intestine. This type of medication is valuable for a patient whose stomach would otherwise not be able to tolerate the drug.

Epistaxis—Nosebleed.

Esophageal—That having to do with the esophagus.

Esophagus—A muscular canal that reaches from the back of the throat to the stomach and carries food and liquids.

Euthanasia—The act of purposefully ending the life of an individual who has an incurable disease.

Exacerbate—To make more severe or violent.

Expectorant—An agent that promotes the expulsion of mucous from the respiratory tract.

F

Fluid extract—A commercial product made to pharmaceutical specifications to concentrate and preserve the active ingredients of a herb or herbal mixture.

G

Gastric—Pertaining to the stomach.

Gastrointestinal—GI. Pertaining to the stomach and intestines.

Generic—A generic medication contains the same active ingredient as its brand name counterpart. Generics are considered by the U.S. Food and Drug Administration (FDA) to be identical in dose, strength, route of administration, safety, efficacy, and intended use.

Ghat—Broad steps that lead down to a holy river, lake, or pond.

Goloka Vrindavan—The personal abode of Lord Sri Krishna where He resides in His original, two-armed form.

Gout—Hereditary disease characterized by inflammation of the joints. Gout is an acute form of arthritis that can affect joints at any location but usually starts in the knee or foot.

H

Hare Krishna *mantra*—Also referred to as the *maha-mantra*. The prescribed *mantra* to be chanted during this age: Hare Krishna Hare Krishna Krishna Krishna Hare Hare/Hare Rama Hare Rama Rama Rama Hare Hare.

Harinama Chadar—A cotton, wool, or silk shawl imprinted with the holy names of Krishna that is worn on the upper part of the body as a wrap.

Hematemesis—Vomiting blood. If the origin is the stomach the color will have a dark "coffee-ground" appearance. If the origin is the pharynx (air passageway from the nasal cavity to the larynx and food passageway from the mouth to the esophagus) it will be bright red in appearance.

Hematuria—Blood in the urine.

Hemorrhoid—Swollen tissue enclosing a mass of dilated veins at the anus, or close to the anus in the rectum.

Hepatocellular carcinoma—A cancerous growth of the liver.

Hepatomegaly—Enlargement of the liver.

Hepatotoxicity—A state of toxic damage to the liver.

Herbal washes—Infusions or diluted tinctures used to bathe wounds, ulcers, or other skin conditions.

Herpetic neuralgia—Nerve pain caused by a herpes infection.
Hormones—Produced from living cells, these substances circulate in body fluids and produce a specific effect on the activity of cells remote from the point of origin.
Hypertension—Higher than normal blood pressure.
Hypoglycemia—An abnormally low concentration of glucose, or sugar, in the blood.
Hypoglycemic—Pertaining to hypoglycemia.
Hypoproteinemia—Abnormally low amount of protein in the blood.
Hypotension—Lower than normal blood pressure.
Hypoxia—Inadequate oxygen supply to the tissues and organs of the body.

I

IV—See "intravenous."
Incontinence—The inability of the body to control the evacuative functions of the bowel and bladder.
Incubation period—The interval of time between exposure to a disease and developing symptoms.
Inflammation—The reaction of body tissue to injury, characterized by pain, heat, redness, and swelling. This can have many causes, including blows, foreign bodies, chemicals, electricity, heat or cold, microorganisms, surgery, or radiation.
Infusion (herbal)—The substance that is obtained by steeping herbs in liquid, without boiling, in order to extract the soluble properties or constituents.
Insulin—A hormone secreted by the pancreas that is important for metabolizing sugar and for maintaining appropriate blood sugar levels.
Intracranial pressure—Pressure within the cranium or skull.
Intravenous—IV. Literally means within or into a vein. A plastic catheter is placed into the vein and left for easy access for fluids, medications, and nutrition.

J

Japa beads—*Japa-mala*; a string of 108 beads, usually made of *tulasi* wood, used to count repetitions of the Hare Krishna *maha-mantra* while chanting.

Jaundice—A condition in which the skin, whites of the eyes, and mucous membranes become yellowish. This condition may be caused by several factors, and is due to an excess amount of a substance called bilirubin in the blood.

K

Kali-yuga—The material creation cycles through a repeating series of four *yugas*, or ages, each characterized by different degrees of piety and spiritual realization. We are currently living in the *Kali-yuga*, which began approximately 5000 years ago and is considered to be the age of quarrel and disturbance.

Karatals—Hand cymbals played in *kirtans* and *bhajans*.

Karma—The force generated by a person's activities; a reaction for each action, good or bad.

Kcal—Kilocalorie; also called a large calorie and abbreviated Cal. A unit measuring the amount of energy a certain amount of food will produce.

Kidney dialysis—A treatment that is used when a person's kidneys are not functioning properly. Blood is passed through a membrane in the dialysis machine; liquid and chemicals are removed that would normally be removed by the kidneys.

Kirtan—Chanting aloud devotional *mantras* and prayers with melody and musical accompaniment.

Krishna—The Supreme Personality of Godhead.

Krishnaloka (Goloka)—The personal abode of Lord Sri Krishna where He resides in His original two-armed form. The topmost planet in the spiritual world.

L

Lactose intolerance—Inability to digest milk products marked by gastrointestinal symptoms due to a deficiency of lactase (an enzyme needed for the absorption of lactose).

Lord Vishnu—An expansion of Krishna who creates and maintains the material universe.

Lumbar puncture—Spinal puncture, made by inserting a needle into the space in the spinal cord at the lumbar (lower area) of the back. Fluid can then be removed for diagnostic purposes, or medication can be injected for anesthesia.

Lymphatic—A network of vessels similar to veins that carry fluids from the tissues back to the blood vessels.

Lymphedema—Edema caused by obstruction of the lymphatics.

Lymph nodes—Rounded bodies consisting of lymphatic tissue that are found at different locations along the lymphatic network. They are found individually or in groups and vary in size from a pinhead to an olive. Their function is to produce lymphocytes and monocytes (large white blood cells) and to filter substances such as bacteria from entering the blood stream.

Lymphocytes—White blood cells that originate in the bone marrow and become mature and functional in lymph organs.

M

Maceration—The softening and breaking down of skin resulting from prolonged exposure to moisture, as in a wound.

Maceration (herbal)—The process of soaking an herb in cool fluid to produce infusions or decoctions.

Mammography—A radiographic study of the breast that is used to diagnose breast cancer.

Mastectomy—Surgical removal of the breast.

Metabolic—Pertaining to metabolism.

Metabolism—The transformation of chemical energy from food eaten into mechanical energy or heat for use by the body.

Metastasis—The movement of cancer cells from one body part or organ to another not directly connected to it.

Myelin sheath—A substance composed of fats and proteins that surrounds the ends of some nerves.

Myocardial infarction—Heart attack; a condition caused by a blockage of one or more of the heart's arteries.

Myocarditis—Inflammation of the walls of the heart, which can be associated with a number of conditions including carbon monoxide poisoning, burns, heat stroke, and infections.

N

Narcotic—A class of drug which depresses the central nervous system and, when administered correctly, relieves pain.

Nasal cannula—Plastic tubing leading from an oxygen tank to the patient with two small outlet prongs that are inserted into the nostrils in order to deliver oxygen at a continuous rate.

Nebulizer—A small device that produces a fine spray or mist. Medication can be added to the container along with normal saline or water, and the contents slowly inhaled by the patient.

Needle biopsy—A needle is inserted into a questionable lesion and a portion of its contents is collected for diagnosis.

Nephropathy—Disease of one or both kidneys.

Neuropathy—Disease of the nerves.

Neurotransmitters—Substances that transmit nerve impulses across a synapse (the point at which a nervous impulse passes from one neuron to another).

O

Opioid—A class of drug that is not derived from opium but has some of the characteristics of opiate narcotics.

Opportunistic infections—Due to the weakened physical state of the patient (usually due to illness), organisms (especially fungi and bacteria) are afforded the opportunity to invade and/or spread with ease, whereas in an otherwise healthy individual they would be defeated by the body's defense mechanisms.

Oral—Pertaining to the mouth.

P

Palliative—The use of medical interventions to lessen the severity of pain or other symptoms without attempting a cure.

Peptic ulcer—An ulcer in the lower end of the esophagus, stomach, or small intestine.

Peripheral neuropathy—Disease of the nerves outside of the brain and spinal cord.

Peripheral nervous system—The part of the nervous system outside of the central nervous system (brain and spinal cord).

Peripheral vascular disease—Disease of the arteries and veins of the extremities (arms and legs) that interferes with the adequate flow of blood to or from the extremities.

Phlebitis—Inflammation of a vein, characterized by pain along the path of the vein, discoloration of the skin, and swelling below the site.

Platelet—A tiny, round, flat disk found in the blood that plays an important role in blood coagulation. Platelets form the thick covering, or scab, that stops the blood flow from an injured vessel.

Polydipsia—Excessive thirst.

Polyphagia—Eating abnormally large amounts of food.

Polyuria—Passing abnormally large amounts of urine.

Prabhupada—The Founder-*acarya* (spiritual leader) of the International Society for Krishna Consciousness (ISKCON).

Prasadam—Food or other articles that have been offered with devotion to Lord Krishna. The "Lord's mercy."

Puja—An offering of worship.

Pujari—A *brahmana* priest who offers *puja*, or worship, to the Deities on the altar.

Pulmonary—Pertaining to the lungs.

Pulmonary function tests—A variety of tests that show the ability of the lungs to take in oxygen and get rid of carbon dioxide. They measure the amount of air that can be exhaled and inhaled as well as the time it takes to exhale.

Pursed-lip breathing—A breathing technique used mostly by persons with chronic lung disease. The lips are positioned like the closure of a draw-string purse to allow air to escape slowly on exhale. This keeps the air sacs of the lung from collapsing.

R

RNA—See "ribonucleic acid."

Rectal—Pertaining to the rectum, which is the lower part of the large intestine. It is about five inches long and is located just before the anal canal.

Respite—A period of time for rest or relief.

Retinopathy—A disorder of the retina (interior lining of the eye).

Rheumatic fever—A systemic (involving the whole body) fever producing disease that can vary in severity, duration, and subsequent problems. Often this illness is followed by serious heart or kidney disease. The cause is unknown, but the onset follows a streptococcal infection.

Ribonucleic acid—RNA. A nucleic acid (substance found in the cells of all living things) that controls the production of protein.

S

Sadhana bhakti—Regulative devotional service that one performs in the beginning stages of spiritual life.

Satiety—A feeling of being full.

Sannyasa—The renounced order of life. The last of the Vedic social orders.

Sannyasi—A person in the renounced Vedic social order.

Sclerosis—A hardening of an organ or body tissue.

Sedation—A state of calm or sleep brought about by the administration of a sedative drug, or a side effect of a drug administered for another reason.

Sitz bath—A basin/tub in which one sits for therapeutic purposes.

Sraddha—A ritual performed to pay homage to one's ancestors.

Srimad Bhagavatam—A history written by Vyasadeva (an incarnation of Lord Krishna) containing eighteen thousand verses in twelve cantos. It was spoken 5000 years ago by Sukadeva Goswami to Pariksit Maharaja, and reveals the essence of pure devotional service to the Lord.

Steatorrhea—Fatty stools due to impaired absorption.

Stenosis—A narrowing of the inner diameter of a passage in the body or orifice, such as a vein, artery, or esophagus.

Subcutaneous—Relating to the area beneath the skin.

Suppository—A semisolid substance, commonly cylindrical or cone shaped, that is introduced into the rectum or vagina where it dissolves and the medication is absorbed.

T

Tachycardia—An abnormally rapid heart rate; usually defined in adults as a heart rate over 100 beats per minute.

Tachypnea—Abnormally rapid respirations, usually defined in adults as over 40 breaths per minute.

Thrombocytopenia—Abnormally low count of platelets in the blood.

Thrush—An infection characterized by white patches and ulcers in the mouth and caused by an overpopulation of Candida albicans (a yeast-like fungus), which is part of the normal flora. A common cause of this overgrowth is the use of antibiotics.

Tilak—Holy clay used to mark the body and forehead of one who is dedicating his life to serving the Lord.

Tincture—A medicinal solution in which alcohol is the solvent.

Tolerance—Drug tolerance is a progressive decrease in the drug's effectiveness.

Toxicity—The degree to which a substance is poisonous.

Trachea—A cartilaginous tube that connects the larynx (area just below the root of the tongue) to the bronchi (main branches to the lungs).

Tulasi-devi—A pure devotee of Lord Krishna in the form of the auspicious *tulasi* plant.

U

Ultrasound—High frequency inaudible sound that is passed through body tissues and organs and viewed on special equipment.

V

Vaishnava—A devotee of Lord Krishna.

Vascular constriction—A constriction of any of the blood or lymph vessels in the body.

Vertigo—A feeling of moving around in space or of things moving about one's self. Sometimes expressed as dizziness or lightheadedness.

Visceral—Pertaining to the internal organs of the body.

Vrindavan—A tract of land in India 135 km south of Delhi where Lord Krishna appeared 5000 years ago.

Y

Yuga—An age of time in the material universe. There are four *yugas* which occur in a repeating cycle. We are currently living in *kali-yuga*, which began approximately 5000 years ago with the departure of Lord Krishna from this planet.

BIBLIOGRAPHY

Active Listening Techniques. (1995).
Phoenix: Community Hospice Training Manual.

Alzheimer's Association
www.alz.org/

American Cancer Society
www.cancer.org/

American Heart Association
www.americanheart.org/

American Medical Association (AMA) *Health Insight*
www.ama-assn.org/

The Basics of Hospice. (1995).
Phoenix: Community Hospice Training Manual.

Bhaktivedanta Swami Prabhupada. (1972). *Bhagavad-gita As It Is.*
New York: The Macmillan Company.

Bhaktivedanta Swami Prabhupada. (1982). *The Nectar of Devotion.*
Los Angeles: Bhaktivedanta Book Trust.

Bhaktivedanta Swami Prabhupada. (1978-1984).
Srimad Bhagavatam of Krsna-Dvaipayana Vyasa. Cantos 1-12.
Los Angeles: Bhaktivedanta Book Trust.

Bhaktivedanta Swami Prabhupada. (1987). *Letters from Srila Prabhupada.*
Los Angeles: Vaishnava Institute.

Body Language- Attitudes Communicated Non verbally. (1995).
Phoenix: Community Hospice Training Manual.
Buckman, Robert, Dr. (1990). *How to Talk to Someone Who's Dying.*
Phoenix: Community Hospice Training Manual.

Carpenter, Donna, O. (Ed.). (1999). *Nurse's Handbook of Alternative and Complementary Therapies.* Springhouse: Springhouse, PA

Centers for Disease Control and Prevention
www.cdc.gov /ncidod/ diseases/hepatitis/a/fact.htm

Clayman, Charles, B., M.D. (Ed.). (1994). *The American Medical Association Family Medical Guide.* New York: Random House, Inc.

The Complete Guide to Natural Healing
New York: International Masters Publishing, Inc.

Czillinger, Ken, Fr. (1997). *How to Help the Dying and Grieving.* Catholic Update. November, 1977.

Dehydration. (1995).
Phoenix: Community Hospice Training Manual.

Directory of Herbs
http:/ /hortweb.cas.psu.edu/vegcrops/herbs.html

The Dying Person's Bill of Rights (1995).
Phoenix: Community Hospice Training Manual.

Everett, Janalee, H., Rev. *Saying Goodbye.* (1995).
Phoenix: Community Hospice Training Manual.

Ferrell-Torry, AT and OJ. Glick. (1993). *The Use of Therapeutic Massage- as a Nursing Intervention to Modify Anxiety and the Perception of Cancer Pain." Cancer Nursing,* April, 1993.

Four Steps to Effective Listening. (1995).
Phoenix: Community Hospice Training Manual.
Friel, Maire, RN., M.N. and Claire B. Tehan, M.A. (1995).
Counteracting Burn-Out for the Hospice Caregiver:
Phoenix: Community Hospice Training Manual.

Grief, Mourning, and Bereavement. (1995).
Phoenix: Community Hospice Training Manual.

Helping the Bereaved After the Funeral. (1995).
Phoenix: Community Hospice Training Manual.

Herb Facts
http:/ /www.herbfacts.com/ index.html

Herbal Information Center
http:/ / www.kcweb.com/herb/herbmain

Hospice Education Institute
www.hospiceworld.org/

Hospice Foundation of America
www.hospicefoundation.org/

How Grief Goes Wrong. (1995).
Phoenix: Community Hospice Training Manual.

Indradyumna Swami. (2001).
Diary of a Traveling Preacher, Volume 3, Chapter 30.

Johns Hopkins Information Website
www.hopkins-id.edu

Karnes, Barbara, *Gone From My Sight-The Dying Experience.*

Kaye, Peter, Dr. (1995). *Notes on Symptom Control in Hospice and Palliative Care.* Essex: Hospice Education Institute.

Kelley, Patricia and Maggie Callahan. (1986). *Is This Confusion, or a Special Communication of the Dying?*
Larson, Dale, G., Ph.D., *Helper Secrets: Invisible Stressors in Hospice Work.*

Loeb, Stanley (Ed.) (1988). *Diseases and Disorders Handbook.* Springhouse: Springhouse Corporation.

Loeb, Stanley (Ed.) (1994). *Handbook of Medical-Surgical Nursing.* Springhouse: Springhouse Corporation

Mayo Foundation for Medical Education and Research
Mayoclinic.com

McCaffery, Margo, RN, MS, FAAN, (1995). *Pain: Assessment and Intervention in Clinical Practice.* Seminar Notes, Spring, 1995.

McCaffery, Margo, RN, MS, FAAN, (1980). *Relieving Pain with Noninvasive Techniques. Nursing 80,* December, 1980.

McIntier, M. Teresa Sister *Experiencing a Terminal Illness.*
Phoenix: Community Hospice Training Manual.

McMahon, Kathleen, RN, MEd, MA, (2000). *Clinical Management of HIV Disease in Adults—in the HAART Era. Nursing Spectrum,* May 15, 2000, 16-18.

McMahon, Kathleen, RN, MEd, MA, ACRN, (2000). *Guided Imagery-A Powerful Therapeutic Support*. Nursing Spectrum, December 11, 2000, 15-17.

'The Most Common Opportunistic Infections.' (1995).
Phoenix: Community Hospice Training Manual.

Musella, Michele, RN, MSN (2000). Making Sense of Scents. *Nursing Spectrum*, April 17, 2000, 22-23.

National Hospice Care Month. (October 30, 2000). *Nursing Spectrum*, 25.
National Multiple Sclerosis Society
www.nmss.org/

The National Parkinson Foundation, Inc.
www.parkinson.org/

National Stroke Association
www.stroke.org/

Ody, Penelope. (1993). *The Complete Medicinal Herbal*
New York: DK Publishing, Inc.

Parkinson's Disease Foundation
www.parkinsons-foundation.org/

Polak, Meraida, BSN, RN and Linda Boynton De Sepulveda, PhD, RN, CRNP. (2000) *Care of the Patient with Amyotrophic Lateral Sclerosis*. Advance for Nurses, May 8, 2000, 15-16

Preparing for Approaching Death. (1995).
Phoenix: Community Hospice Training Manual.

Redding, Beverlee, E. (1986), *Nursing Manual of Hospice Care*.

Redwood, Daniel. (1997), *Interview with Elisabeth Kubler-Ross, M.D.-On Death and Dying*. http://www.doubleclickd.com/kubler.html.

Scott, Abigail. (2000). *Ensuring Fair Care and Compassion at the End of Life. Advance for Nurses*, April 24, 2000, 27, 32.

Servodidio, Cammille A., RN, MPH, CRNO and Ellen Williams, RN, MA. *Identifying Pain in the Hospice Patient*. Nursing Spectrum, July 24, 2000, 18-20.

Stoddard, San dol. (1991), *The Hospice Movement.* New York: Vintage Books.

Storey, Porter, M.D. (1994). *Primer of Palliative Care.* Gainesville: The Academy of Hospice Physicians.

"Survival Time of Terminally Ill Overestimated." (March 20, 2000). *Nursing Spectrum,* 27.

Thomas, Clayton, Lay. (Ed.). (1993). *Taber's Cyclopedic Medical Dictionary.* Philadelphia: F.A. Davis Company.

Weathersby, Trudy. (2000). *Death and Dying.* http://dying.about.com/health/dying/library/weekly/aa072897.htm

Zerwekh, Joyce V., EdD, MA, BSN. (1997). *Do Dying Patients Really Need IV Fluids?"* www.ajn.org/

Zerwekh, Joyce V., RNC, MA. (1983). *The Dehydration Question. Nursing '83 Magazine,* January, 1983, 47-51.